Carol L. Jenkins, MPA, PhD
Editor

Widows and Divorcees in Later Life: On Their Own Again

Widows and Divorcees in Later Life: On Their Own Again has been co-published simultaneously as *Journal of Women & Aging,* Volume 15, Numbers 2/3 2003.

More pre-publication
REVIEWS, COMMENTARIES, EVALUATIONS . . .

"**A**ddresses a wide range of issues facing women in later life, including physical and mental health, economic security, and family support. Great attention is paid to the variety of women's experiences with chapters dealing with minority women in the United States as well as the Philippines, Fiji, Kenya, England, and Wales. I especially appreciated the book's attention to the lives of African women.

Christine L. Himes, PhD
Associate Professor of Psychology
Syracuse University

"**I**nformative and stimulating. . . . By the time I finished reading this text, I was already begining to think of ways to incorporate some of the findings into my own program of research. The contributing authors were obviously carefully selected for the quality of their work and the unique contributions they could make to the overall organization and relevance of the text."

Shirley S. Travis, PhD, APRN, BC, Dean W. Colvard Distinguished Professor
College of Health and Human Services
University of North Carolina at Charlotte

The Haworth Press, Inc.

Widows and Divorcees in Later Life: On Their Own Again

Widows and Divorcees in Later Life: On Their Own Again has been co-published simultaneously as *Journal of Women & Aging*, Volume 15, Numbers 2/3 2003.

The *Journal of Women & Aging* Monographic "Separates"

Below is a list of "separates," which in serials librarianship means a special issue simultaneously published as a special journal issue or double-issue *and* as a "separate" hardbound monograph. (This is a format which we also call a "DocuSerial.")

"Separates" are published because specialized libraries or professionals may wish to purchase a specific thematic issue by itself in a format which can be separately cataloged and shelved, as opposed to purchasing the journal on an on-going basis. Faculty members may also more easily consider a "separate" for classroom adoption.

"Separates" are carefully classified separately with the major book jobbers so that the journal tie-in can be noted on new book order slips to avoid duplicate purchasing.

You may wish to visit Haworth's website at . . .

http://www.HaworthPress.com

. . . to search our online catalog for complete tables of contents of these separates and related publications.

You may also call 1-800-HAWORTH (outside US/Canada: 607-722-5857), or Fax 1-800-895-0582 (outside US/Canada: 607-771-0012), or e-mail at:

docdelivery@haworthpress.com

Widows and Divorcees in Later Life: On Their Own Again, edited by Carol L. Jenkins, MPA, PhD (Vol. 15, No.2/3, 2003). *"Exhaustive. . . . Richly textured. . . . This book may well emerge as a seminal work on this topic."* (David K. Brown, PhD, Associate Director, Center on Aging, West Virginia University)

Health Expectations for Older Women: International Perspectives, edited by Sarah B. Laditka, PhD (Vol. 14, No. 1/2, 2002). *"Brings together noted experts from around the world who shed new light on how women age. . . . This volume is sweeping in its coverage, including specific analyses of the U.S., the U.K., Japan, Canada, The Netherlands, and Fiji, as well as an overview of all 191 WHO member countries. A nice balance of country-specific and global studies. . . . Gerontologists, epidemiologists, and demographers will find the information presented to be timely, rigorous, and accessible."* (Christine L. Himes, PhD, Associate Professor of Sociology, Syracuse University)

Fundamentals of Feminist Gerontology, edited by J. Dianne Garner, DSW (Vol. 11, No. 2/3, 1999). *Strives to increase women's self-esteem and their overall quality of life by encouraging education and putting a stop to age, sex, and race discrimination.*

Old, Female, and Rural, edited by B. Jan McCulloch (Vol. 10, No. 4, 1998). *"An excellent job of bringing together experts from four different disciplines to illuminate the basic interdisciplinary nature of gerontology."* (Dr. Jean Turner, Associate Professor, Human Development and Family Services, University of Arkansas, Fayetteville, Arkansas)

Relationships Between Women in Later Life, edited by Karen A. Roberto (Vol. 8, No. 3/4, 1996). *"Provides an impressive array of issues about women's social networks. . . . Important, up-to-date empirical studies that will fill a significant gap in our understanding about the great diversity in the lives of older women today."* (European Federation of the Elderly)

Older Women with Chronic Pain, edited by Karen A. Roberto (Vol. 6, No. 4, 1994). *"Readers interested in the health concerns of older women, and older women themselves, will appreciate the insight and information in this book."* (Feminist Bookstore News)

Women and Healthy Aging: Living Productively in Spite of It All, edited by J. Dianne Garner and Alice A. Young (Vol. 5, No. 3/4, 1994). *"For those who are not aged themselves, it helps to bring about insights that are not possible when one holds the commonly taught view that disability of any degree is strictly debilitating."* (Linda Vinton, PhD, Associate Professor, School of Social Work, Florida State University; Research Affiliate, Pepper Institute on Aging and Public Policy)

Women in Mid-Life: Planning for Tomorrow, edited by Christopher L. Hayes (Vol. 4, No. 4, 1993). *"Contains illuminating insights into aspects of women's mid-life experiences." (Age and Ageing)*

Women, Aging and Ageism, edited by Evelyn Rosenthal (Vol. 2, No. 2, 1990). *"Readers should find this book helpful in gaining new insights to issues women face in old age. . . . Enlightening." (Educational Gerontology)*

Women as They Age: Challenge, Opportunity, and Triumph, edited by J. Dianne Garner and Susan O. Mercer (Vol. 1, No. 1/2/3, 1989). *"Offers provocative insights into the strengths, dilemmas, and challenges confronting the current and future cohorts of older women." (Affilia: Journal of Women and Social Work)*

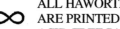

Widows and Divorcees in Later Life: On Their Own Again

Carol L. Jenkins, MPA, PhD
Editor

Widows and Divorcees in Later Life: On Their Own Again has been co-published simultaneously as *Journal of Women & Aging*, Volume 15, Numbers 2/3 2003.

The Haworth Press, Inc.
New York • London • Oxford

Published by

Harrington Park Press®, 10 Alice Street, Binghamton, NY 13904-1580 USA

Harrington Park Press® is an imprint of The Haworth Press, Inc., 10 Alice Street, Binghamton, NY 13904-1580 USA.

Widows and Divorcees in Later Life : On Their Own Again has been co-published simultaneously as *Journal of Women & Aging*™, Volume 15, Numbers 2/3 2003.

The development, preparation, and publication of this work has been undertaken with great care. However, the publisher, employees, editors, and agents of The Haworth Press and all imprints of The Haworth Press, Inc., including The Haworth Medical Press® and Pharmaceutical Products Press®, are not responsible for any errors contained herein or for consequences that may ensue from use of materials or information contained in this work. Opinions expressed by the author(s) are not necessarily those of The Haworth Press, Inc. With regard to case studies, identities and circumstances of individuals discussed herein have been changed to protect confidentiality. Any resemblance to actual persons, living or dead, is entirely coincidental.

Cover design by Jennifer M. Gaska

Library of Congress Cataloging-in-Publication Data

Widows and divorcees in later life : on their own again / Carol L. Jenkins, editor.
    p. cm.
    "Co-published simultaneously as Journal of women & aging, Volume 15, Numbers 2/3."
    Includes bibliographical references and index.
    ISBN 0-7890-2191-9 (cloth : alk. paper) – ISBN 0-7890-2192-7 (pbk. : alk. paper)
    1. Widows–United States. 2. Divorced women–United States. 3. Aged women–United States. I. Jenkins, Carol Lynn. II. Journal of women & aging.
HQ1058.5.U5W53 2003
305.48'9653–dc21
                                                 2003009785

Indexing, Abstracting & Website/Internet Coverage

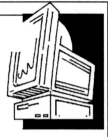

This section provides you with a list of major indexing & abstracting services. That is to say, each service began covering this periodical during the year noted in the right column. Most Websites which are listed below have indicated that they will either post, disseminate, compile, archive, cite or alert their own Website users with research-based content from this work. (This list is as current as the copyright date of this publication.)

Abstracting, Website/Indexing Coverage . . . . Year When Coverage Began

- *Abstracts in Anthropology* **1992**
- *Abstracts in Social Gerontology: Current Literature on Aging* **1988**
- *Academic ASAP <www.galegroup.com>* **1992**
- *Academic Index (on-line)* **1992**
- *Academic Search Elite (EBSCO)* **1996**
- *AgeInfo CD-ROM* **1995**
- *AgeLine Database* **1990**
- *Behavioral Medicine Abstracts* **1992**
- *Cambridge Scientific Abstracts (Health & Safety Science Abstracts)*
  <www.csa.com> **1993**
- *CINAHL (Cumulative Index to Nursing & Allied Health*
  Literature), in print, EBSCO, and SilverPlatter, Data-Star, and
  PaperChase. (Support materials include Subject Heading List,
  Database Search Guide, and Instructional Video)
  <www.cinahl.com> **1997**
- *CNPIEC Reference Guide: Chinese National Directory*
  of Foreign Periodicals **1995**
- *Combined Health Information Database (CHID)* **1995**
- *Contemporary Women's Issues* **1998**

(continued)

- *Current Contents/Social & Behavioral Sciences
  <www.isinet.com>* 1995
- *e-psyche, LLC <www.e-psyche.net.* 2003
- *Expanded Academic ASAP <www.galegroup.com>* 1992
- *Family & Society Studies Worldwide
  <www.nisc.com>* 1996
- *Family Violence & Sexual Assault Bulletin* 1999
- *Feminist Periodicals: A Current Listing of Contents* 1989
- *GenderWatch <www.slinfo.com>* 1999
- *Guide to Social Science & Religion in Periodical Literature* 1992
- *Human Resources Abstracts (HRA)* 1992
- *IBZ International Bibliography of Periodical Literature
  <www.saur.de>* 1996
- *Index Guide to College Journals (core list compiled by
  integrating 48 indexes frequently used to support
  undergraduate programs in small to medium sized
  libraries)* 1999
- *Index Medicus (National Library of Medicine)
  <www.nlm.nih.gov>* 1999
- *Index to Periodical Articles Related to Law* 1992
- *MasterFILE: Updated database from EBSCO Publishing* 1996
- *MEDLINE (National Library of Medicine) <www.nlm.nih.gov>* 1999
- *National Center for Chronic Disease Prevention & Health
  Promotion (NCCDPHP)* 1998
- *National Clearinghouse for Primary Care Information
  (NCPCI)* 1995
- *New Literature on Old Age* 1995
- *Periodical Abstracts, Research II (broad coverage indexing &
  abstracting database from University Microfilms International
  [UMI] 300 North Zeeb Road, P.O. Box 1346,
  Ann Arbor, MI 48106-1346)* 1992
- *Periodical Abstracts Select (abstracting & indexing service
  covering most frequently requested journals in general
  reference, plus journals requested in libraries serving
  undergraduate programs, available from University Microfilms International [UMI], 300 North Zeeb Road,
  P.O. Box 1346, Ann Arbor, MI 48106-1346)* 1994

(continued)

- *Physiotherapy Evidence Database (PEDro) . . . Internet-based database of: a) articles describing evidence-based clinical trials in physiotherapy; b) systematic reviews of each; c) single-case experimental studies of efficacy of therapeutic interventions <www.pedro.fhs.usyd.edu.au>* **2003**
- *Psychological Abstracts (PsycINFO) <www.apa.org>* **2001**
- *RESEARCH ALERT/ISI Alerting Services <www.isinet.com>* **1995**
- *Social Sciences Citation Index <www.isinet.com>* **1995**
- *Social Scisearch <www.isinet.com>* **1995**
- *Social Services Abstracts <www.csa.com>* **1992**
- *Social Work Abstracts <www.silverplatter.com/catalog/swab.htm>* . . . **1992**
- *Sociological Abstracts (SA) <www.csa.com>* **1992**
- *Studies on Women Abstracts <www.tandf.co.uk>* **1988**
- *SwetsNet <www.swetsnet.com>* **2001**
- *Women Studies Abstracts* **1991**
- *Women's Healthbeat* **1999**
- *Women's Studies Index (Indexed Comprehensively)* **1992**

Special Bibliographic Notes related to special journal issues (separates) and indexing/abstracting:

- indexing/abstracting services in this list will also cover material in any "separate" that is co-published simultaneously with Haworth's special thematic journal issue or DocuSerial. Indexing/abstracting usually covers material at the article/chapter level.
- monographic co-editions are intended for either non-subscribers or libraries which intend to purchase a second copy for their circulating collections.
- monographic co-editions are reported to all jobbers/wholesalers/approval plans. The source journal is listed as the "series" to assist the prevention of duplicate purchasing in the same manner utilized for books-in-series.
- to facilitate user/access services all indexing/abstracting services are encouraged to utilize the co-indexing entry note indicated at the bottom of the first page of each article/chapter/contribution.
- this is intended to assist a library user of any reference tool (whether print, electronic, online, or CD-ROM) to locate the monographic version if the library has purchased this version but not a subscription to the source journal.
- individual articles/chapters in any Haworth publication are also available through the Haworth Document Delivery Service (HDDS).

ABOUT THE EDITOR

Carol L. Jenkins, MPA, PhD, is Associate Professor of Social Work and teaches courses in the gerontology programs through the Center on Aging, East Carolina University. She has previously held positions as Assistant Professor of Health Administration, University of North Carolina at Charlotte; Assistant Professor of Public Administration and Health Administration, Auburn University; and Research Associate, Center for Policy Research, The Maxwell School, Syracuse University. Dr. Jenkins' research interests focus on long-term care arrangement decisions, disability measurement, caregiver stress, and supportive programs for caregivers. She is currently studying the implementation and effectiveness of the National Family Caregiver Support Program. Her research has been published in numerous journals, including *Journal of Women & Aging, Policy Studies Review, Journal of Aging & Social Policy, Administration and Policy in Mental Health,* and *Home Health Care Services Quarterly.*

Widows and Divorcees in Later Life: On Their Own Again

CONTENTS

Introduction: Widows and Divorcees in Later Life   1
Carol L. Jenkins, MPA, PhD

Increased Hospitalization Risk for Recently Widowed
Older Women and Protective Effects of Social Contacts   7
James N. Laditka, DA, PhD
Sarah B. Laditka, PhD

Health, Widowhood, and Family Support in the North
and South Pacific: A Comparative Study   29
James W. McNally, PhD

African Widows: Anthropological and Historical Perspectives   49
Maria G. Cattell, PhD

The Impact of Minority Group Status on the Projected
Retirement Income of Divorced Women
in the Baby Boom Cohort   67
Barbara A. Butrica, PhD
Howard M. Iams, PhD

Gender, Widowhood, and Long-Term Care in the Older Mexican
American Population   89
Jacqueline L. Angel, PhD
Nora Douglas
Ronald J. Angel, PhD

Transitions to Supported Environments in England
   and Wales Among Elderly Widowed and Divorced Women:
   The Changing Balance Between Co-Residence with Family
   and Institutional Care   107
     Karen Glaser, PhD
     Emily Grundy, PhD
     Kevin Lynch, BSc

Care Arrangement Choices for Older Widows:
   Decision Participants' Perspectives   127
     Carol L. Jenkins, MPA, PhD

Widowhood and Spirituality: Coping Responses
   to Bereavement   145
     Scott T. Michael, PhD
     Martha R. Crowther, PhD
     Bettina Schmid, MA
     Rebecca S. Allen, PhD

Not on Their Own Again: Psychological, Social,
   and Health Characteristics of Custodial African
   American Grandmothers   167
     Dorothy S. Ruiz, PhD
     Carolyn W. Zhu, PhD
     Martha R. Crowther, PhD, MPH

Conclusions   185
     Carol L. Jenkins, MPA, PhD

About the Contributors   189

Index   193

Introduction:
Widows and Divorcees in Later Life

Carol L. Jenkins, MPA, PhD

Older women have been of interest to academics and researchers from a wide array of disciplines for many years. One reason for this is their larger representation in the older population. They outnumber men within the population that is over 65 years of age. And they become an ever larger proportion of the older population as we consider the middle-old and old-old age groups: more than two of every three people over 75 years of age are women, and nearly four of every five people over 85 are women (Social Security Administration, 1998).

Another reason for the interest in older women is that they face many problems as they age, some of which are gender related. Older people in general face a higher likelihood of increasing disability, especially at older ages. Because women have longer life expectancies than men, however, they are likely to spend a longer period of time coping with disability and in need of assistance with normal activities of daily living (ADLs). Older women are more likely than men to face threats to their economic security. Those women who have worked during their lifetime have often earned less which reduces their ability to save for retirement and results in lower Social Security benefits; they are also less likely than men to have pension income. Many older women live alone which further reduces their access to familial caregiving and economic

[Haworth co-indexing entry note]: "Introduction: Widows and Divorcees in Later Life." Jenkins, Carol L. Co-published simultaneously in *Journal of Women & Aging* (The Haworth Press, Inc.) Vol. 15, No. 2/3, 2003, pp. 1-6; and: *Widows and Divorcees in Later Life: On Their Own Again* (ed: Carol L. Jenkins) The Haworth Press, Inc., 2003, pp. 1-6. Single or multiple copies of this article are available for a fee from The Haworth Document Delivery Service [1-800-HAWORTH, 9:00 a.m. - 5:00 p.m. (EST). E-mail address: docdelivery@haworthpress.com].

resources. Older women also tend to have more difficulty with chronic health problems than older men, thus increasing their need for ongoing assistance with ADL difficulties.

Adding to these problems is society's view and treatment of older people in general, but women in particular. They have lost both youth and physical attractiveness, which are primary factors in assigning value to women. They are past childbearing, another means of providing value to society. Thus, many women face old age without the perceived extrinsic value and resources necessary for a secure and comfortable lifestyle.

FOCUS ON OLDER WIDOWS AND DIVORCEES

The previously discussed problems may be magnified for older women who are widowed or divorced. Women are more likely to be widowed due to their longer life expectancies and the propensity of men to marry younger women; about half of women over 65 were widows in 1997 (U.S. Census Bureau, 1998). While the numbers of divorced women in the current older population is relatively small, this is likely to change. Divorce rates have increased in the latter part of the 20th century, particularly for mid-life women so there are likely to be more divorcees in future cohorts (Choi, 1992).

Economic well-being. While older women are more likely to be poor than older men, the problem is particularly acute for women without a spouse. Those women who have not worked are dependent in their later years on their spouse's lifetime earning record. Upon the loss of their spouse, their income can be dramatically reduced due to lower Social Security benefits and loss of pension income. Three of every four older poor individuals are women, with women being twice as likely to be living in poverty as men (Smeeding, 1999; Choudhury & Leonesio, 1997). Poverty rates are highest for unmarried (i.e., widowed, divorced, and never married) women, however: 20% are living in poverty compared to only 5% of married women. Widows and divorcees have significantly longer periods of poverty than married women (Vartanian & McNamara, 2002) and thus have a reduced likelihood of exiting from poverty (Dodge, 1995). It is well established that it is the loss of a spouse and his economic resources that is associated with declines in the economic well-being of widows (e.g., Burkhauser, Butler, & Holden, 1991; Zick & Smith, 1991). At the same time, it appears that divorcees face the greatest risk of poverty in old age (Choi, 1992).

Living arrangements. An older woman's living situation has much to do with her ability to avoid poverty and to freely access assistance with ADLs. Living alone is associated with a higher likelihood of poverty (Hardy & Hazelrigg, 1993), while co-residence with other family members often allows a poor older woman to move out of poverty (Dodge, 1995). Co-resident family members also provide a frail older woman easier and more continuous access to assistance with daily tasks such as transferring in and out of bed, bathing, and dressing. Unfortunately, however, a large majority of widows do not benefit from co-residence: statistics show that about 70% live alone (U.S. Census Bureau, 1998).

Physical health. Much of the research on health effects for older unmarried women is focused on widows. Annual mean health care costs are higher for widows, and highest for those who reported happy marriages. Not surprisingly, the time of greatest risk for health problems is in the first few months following the loss of the spouse (Prigerson, Maciejewski, & Rosenheck, 2000). Mean weight loss and prevalence of weight loss is higher among widows (Shahar, Schultz, Shahar, & Wing, 2001). Widowhood causes loneliness and leads to less interest in activities surrounding eating, including meal planning, shopping, and meal preparation; this eventually leads to weight loss (Rosenbloom & Whittington, 1993). Widows tend to eat more meals alone, eat more commercially prepared meals each week, have less variety in their dietary intake, and eat fewer snacks and homemade meals, sometimes even skipping meals (Quandt, McDonald, Arcury, Bell, & Vitolins, 2000). As a result, their nutritional status declines which contributes to excess morbidity and mortality (Rauscher, 1993). Research has shown that divorce has negative consequences for women's mortality (Smith & Zick, 1994).

Psychological well-being. The loss of a spouse is a major life event. Although people react very differently to such situations, many find it to be a traumatic and life-changing event associated with increased levels of stress. Research shows that the loss of a spouse through death or divorce adversely affects many older women's psychological well-being (Miller & Smerglia, 1998). One-third of widows meet the criteria for clinical depression in the first month after a spouse's death, and half of these remain clinically depressed a year later (National Institute of Mental Health, 1999).

Social support. Social support is particularly important for older widows and divorcees as it helps to mitigate the effects of some of the factors discussed above. Social support, or the perception of available help from one's family, friends, and neighbors, can help to alleviate the physical and psychological effects of loss-related stress (Miller & Smerglia, 1998). There are differences in the effects of social support between widows and divorcees. It may be more important to widows, as there is some evidence that divorcees are more independent (Kitson & Roach, 1989). Those divorcees who desire social support may be less likely to receive it, however, as it has been shown to decrease after a divorce (Krause & Jay, 1991). The type of social support is also important. Having someone listen to personal problems may be more helpful in alleviating divorcees' stress, while practical help (e.g., assistance with transportation, help with house repairs) is more useful in relieving widows' distress (Miller & Smerglia, 1998).

The availability of social support is, of course, the primary factor affecting whether widows and divorcees actually find themselves "on their own again" or not. In a very real sense, they can be considered on their own since they no longer have the partner with whom they have spent a large share of their lifetime and on whom they have counted for many kinds of support. The studies in this book explore the theme of widows and divorcees on their own, and investigate the various ways in which public policies, as well as family members and friends, help to alleviate the adverse effects associated with losing a spouse.

WIDOWS AND DIVORCEES IN LATER LIFE: AN OVERVIEW

As we have seen, older widows and divorcees face many challenges. This volume looks anew at some of the issues discussed above, offering fresh insights into the lives of older widows and divorcees. Laditka and Laditka address the health effects of widowhood as they relate to increased acute care episodes. Recognizing the value of social support, they investigate how widows' social contacts help to protect them from adverse health effects related to the loss of a spouse. How do the impacts of health and widowhood differ for older widows in underdeveloped countries? McNally investigates this topic in a cross-national study in which he compares the levels of family support for older widows in two small island communities within the Philippines and Fiji. His research tests the assumptions of altruism as the basis for providing assistance to older family members that are central to many models investigating long-term care in underdeveloped nations. The focus on non-Western countries continues with Cattell's exploration of widowhood in sub-Saharan Africa. She discusses the various socioeconomic and cultural contexts in which African widows live their lives, with an emphasis on the effects of the AIDS epidemic and poor economic conditions.

We then shift back to the United States to address an important problem for many older women: economic well-being. A large share of the current cohort of older women is poor. There is speculation that this may change for future cohorts since younger women have had more opportunities to obtain advanced education and to participate in the labor market, both of which should increase retirement income. Butrica and Iams address this issue as they investigate projections of retirement income for divorced women in the baby boom cohort, with a focus on the effects of minority group membership.

Long-term care is another important issue facing older women. Since the bulk of such care is provided by family members, widows and divorcees are often at special risk for needing formal long-term care. Several articles address these issues. Angel, Douglas, and Angel consider gender effects on the use of formal services for a sample of older Mexican widows and widowers. Insights into living arrangement transitions among divorced and widowed women in the United Kingdom are provided by Glaser, Grundy, and Lynch. They investigate the propensity of older widows and divorcees to move from independent living to one of two other arrangements: private households and institutions. Jenkins uses qualitative methods to study the long-term care arrangement decision process from the perspectives of each of the decision participants. She identifies themes associated with the decision in general as well as those of specific decision participants.

Michael, Crowther, Schmid, and Allen consider the psychological effects of widowhood and the bereavement process. They review the literature on how religion and spirituality affect widows' ability to cope and identify several areas for future research in this emerging field. In another study related to the psychological well-being of older women, Ruiz, Zhu, and Crowther investigate the indicators of depression among a sample of older custodial African American grandmothers. Far from being "on their own" again, they have taken on responsibility for providing care to their grandchildren.

This volume presents new perspectives on the lives of older widows and divorcees, and on some of the problems they face in adjusting to life without a spouse. We look at these issues through the lens of a life transition from the togetherness of marriage to the solitude of singleness, and explore how older widows and divorcees are adapting to being "on their own again."

REFERENCES

Burkhauser, R.V., Butler, J.S., & Holden, K.C. (1991). How the death of a spouse affects economic wellbeing after retirement: A hazard model approach. *Social Science Quarterly, 72*, 504-519.

Choi, N.G. (1992). Correlates of the economic status of widowed and divorced elderly women. *Journal of Family Issues, 13*, 38-56.

Choudhury, S., & Leonesio, M.V. (1997). Life-cycle aspects of poverty among older women. *Social Security Bulletin, 60*, 17-36.

Dodge, H.H. (1995). Movements out of poverty among elderly widows. *Journal of Gerontology: Social Sciences, 50B*, S240-S249.

Hardy, M.A., & Hazelrigg, L.E. (1993). The gender of poverty in an aging population. *Research on Aging, 15*, 243-278.

Kitson, G.C., & Roach, M.J. (1989). Independence and social and psychological adjustment in widowhood and divorce. In D.A. Lund (Ed.), *Older bereaved spouses: Research with practical applications.* New York: Hemisphere.

Krause, N., & Jay, G. (1991). Stress, social support, and negative interaction in later life. *Research on Aging, 13*, 333-363.

Miller, N.B., & Smerglia, V.L. (1998). Stressful life events, social support, and the distress of widowed and divorced women. *Journal of Family Issues, 19*, 181-204.

National Institute of Mental Health. (1999). The many dimensions of depression in women: Women at risk [Online]. Available: http://www.nimh.nih.gov/depression/women/risk.html.

Prigerson, H.G., Maciejewski, P.K., & Rosenheck, R.A. (2000). Preliminary explorations of the harmful interactive effects of widowhood and marital harmony on health, health service use, and health care costs. *The Gerontologist, 40*, 349-357.

Quandt, S.A., McDonald, J., Arcury, T.A., Bell, R.A., & Vitolins, M.A. (2000). Nutritional self-management of elderly widows in rural communities. *The Gerontologist, 40*, 86-96.

Rauscher, C. (1993). Malnutrition among the elderly. *Canadian Family Physicians, 39*, 1395-1403.

Rosenbloom, C.A., & Whittington, F.J. (1993). The effects of bereavement on eating behaviors and nutrient intakes in elderly widowed persons. *Journal of Gerontology: Social Sciences, 48*, S223-S229.

Shahar, D.R., Schultz, R., Shahar, A., & Wing, R.R. (2001). The effect of widowhood on weight change, dietary intake, and eating behavior in the elderly population. *Journal of Aging & Health, 13*, 186-200.

Smeeding, T.M. (1999). Social security reform: Improving benefit adequacy and economic security for women. Syracuse, NY: Aging Studies Policy Brief #16.

Smith, K.R., & Zick, C.D. (1994). Linked lives, dependent demise? Survival analysis of husbands and wives. *Demography, 31* 81-93.

Social Security Administration. (1998). Fast facts and figures about social security 1998. Office of Research, Evaluation, and Statistics. Washington, DC: U.S. Government Printing Office.

U.S. Census Bureau. (1998). Nearly 70 percent of elderly widows live alone. [Online]. Available: http://www.census.gov/population/www/socdemo/ms-la.html.

Vartanian, T.P., & McNamara, J.M. (2002). Older women in poverty: The impact of midlife factors. *Journal of Marriage & Family, 64*, 532-549.

Zick, C.D., & Smith, K.R. (1991). Patterns of economic change surrounding the death of a spouse. *Journal of Gerontology: Social Sciences, 46*, S310-S320.

Increased Hospitalization Risk
for Recently Widowed Older Women
and Protective Effects of Social Contacts

James N. Laditka, DA, PhD
Sarah B. Laditka, PhD

SUMMARY. This study examines effects of recent widowhood on health for a nationally representative sample of older women in the United States. Mediating effects of social connectedness on the health of recently widowed women are also explored. Using data from the 1984-1990 Longitudinal Study of Aging and Medicare claims, discrete-time hazard models estimate the risk of hospitalization for any 30-day period for women who were married at the time of the baseline survey (n = 1,138). Compared to women who are not recently widowed, those recently widowed have a 40% higher risk of hospitalization. Social connectedness, measured by having phoned a friend/neighbor or family member in the period prior to the baseline survey, significantly decreases hospitalization risk for the recently widowed. The findings indicate that recent widowhood has a large adverse effect on the health of older

Address correspondence to: James N. Laditka, The Arnold School of Public Health, HESC Building, 800 Sumter Street, University of South Carolina, Columbia, SC 29208 (E-mail: jladitka@gwm.sc.edu).

This paper was presented in part at the 30th State Society on Aging of New York Conference, Albany, New York, October 31, 2002.

[Haworth co-indexing entry note]: "Increased Hospitalization Risk for Recently Widowed Older Women and Protective Effects of Social Contacts." Laditka, James N., and Sarah B. Laditka. Co-published simultaneously in *Journal of Women & Aging* (The Haworth Press, Inc.) Vol. 15, No. 2/3, 2003, pp. 7-28; and: *Widows and Divorcees in Later Life: On Their Own Again* (ed: Carol L. Jenkins) The Haworth Press, Inc., 2003, pp. 7-28. Single or multiple copies of this article are available for a fee from The Haworth Document Delivery Service [1-800-HAWORTH, 9:00 a.m. - 5:00 p.m. (EST). E-mail address: docdelivery@haworthpress.com].

women. Results highlight the need to provide additional support to recently widowed older women. *[Article copies available for a fee from The Haworth Document Delivery Service: 1-800-HAWORTH. E-mail address: <docdelivery@haworthpress.com> Website: <http://www.HaworthPress.com> © 2003 by The Haworth Press, Inc. All rights reserved.]*

KEYWORDS. Bereavement, health, hospitalization, widows, social contacts

INTRODUCTION

The United States and many other countries are experiencing unprecedented population aging (Kinsella, 2000). Women live notably longer than men, and the risk of being widowed is over three times greater for older women than for older men (Burkhauser & Smeeding, 1994). Despite these demographic trends, relatively few studies have examined the period of transition for older women after a husband's death. Much of the research in this area has focused on short-term adverse effects of widowhood on physical and psychological well-being, often referred to as bereavement effects (Lillard & Waite, 1995; Korenman, Goldman, & Fu, 1997; Kravdal, 2001; Mendes De Leon, Kasl, & Jacobs, 1994). The majority of these studies have examined bereavement and mortality. In these studies, researchers have largely found that widowed women have significantly higher mortality rates than married women (e.g., Korenman et al., 1997).

This study examines effects of recent and later widowhood on health for a nationally representative sample of older women in the United States. Data are from the United States' Longitudinal Study of Aging. We use hospitalization as an indicator of morbidity. We also explore mediating effects of social connectedness on the health status of recently widowed women. Although our primary analysis focuses on short-term health effects of widowhood, we frame our research in a life cycle perspective. This framework emphasizes individual development throughout the life course. Placing the transition to widowhood in a developmental perspective of life events recognizes the significance of the loss of a spouse for older women. At the same time, this view helps to avoid an exclusively negative perspective of widowhood. The fact that the typical woman can expect to live a notable length of time after her husband's death makes an understanding of short-term adverse effects of widowhood on health important for practitioners and policy makers, caregivers and friends. A fuller understanding of this life event highlights the need to provide assistance to recently widowed older women, to help reduce the risk of short-term negative health events associated with a husband's death.

TRANSITION TO WIDOWHOOD

A small but growing number of researchers suggest that as the number of older women grows throughout the world, the transition to widowhood will become more generally accepted as a normal developmental life cycle phase (Feldman, Byles, & Beaumont, 2000; Porter, 1995). These studies emphasize widowhood is not always an unambiguously negative event. The short-term transition to widowhood is stressful, both physically and psychologically. However, this transition may also be associated with positive features for some older women. For example, some women may experience freedom from caring for a disabled spouse. Others may achieve greater autonomy after many years living with a dominant spouse. Still others may enjoy more fully developed social networks outside the home.

Prior research on the widowhood transition has largely focused on short-term effects of widowhood. Most studies have examined associations between widowhood and mortality. Almost all of these studies have found widowhood is associated with a significantly increased risk of death (Lillard & Waite, 1995; Korenman et al., 1997). The relationship between widowhood and mortality has been found to be stronger for men than for women (Hu & Goldman, 1990; Lillard & Waite, 1995). Among older women who are widowed, this relationship is notably mitigated by greater economic resources (Bound, Duncon, & Oleinick, 1991; Lillard & Waite, 1995).

To our knowledge, only a few studies have examined the relationship between widowhood and morbidity. Using data from the Longitudinal Study of Aging, Goldman, Korenman, and Weinstein (1995) found widowed women were more likely to be disabled, measured by impairments in Activities of Daily Living (ADLs). Using data from the baseline survey of Women's Health Australia (WHA), Byles, Feldman, and Mishra (1999), studied three dimensions: health; financial and practical matters; and social relationships with children, other relatives, and non-relatives. They found that the health of women who were widowed one year or less was significantly poorer than that of women widowed more than a year, or than that of married women. Also using data from the baseline wave of the WHA, Feldman et al. (2000) performed a qualitative analysis of the three dimensions studied by Byles et al. (1999), and found women who had been widowed for two years or less experienced more adverse effects of widowhood than those who had been widowed for more than two years.

In a related area, a number of studies have examined the relationship between social contacts, marital status, and health (Anson, 1989). It is established that the quality and quantity of social supports influences women's well-being much more than that of men, and that women have larger and more diverse social support networks than men (e.g., Antonucci & Akiyama, 1987). Prior research has also found that although social support systems play an important role among recently widowed women and men, there is a great deal of variability in coping measures used by widowed people (Kirschling & McBride, 1989). Two previous studies of widowhood and mortality and/or morbidity have found that health effects of widowhood are attenuated when social controls are included. Goldman and colleagues (1995) examined effects of various social factors, including contact with children or friends and participation in social activities, and found that less participation in social activities was associated with modest increases in disability. Lillard and Waite (1995) concluded that mortality was reduced for widowed women when controls for living arrangements (having another adult residing in the household) and income were included. Umberson (1992) found that women and men who transitioned from married to unmarried were more likely to adopt negative health behaviors than those who remained married. She suggests that higher mortality for people who are widowed may result both from the stress that accompanies loss of a spouse, and from the loss of support from the spouse for lifestyle choices related to health and to use of preventive health services.

Our analysis contributes to the small body of literature examining the relationship between the transition to widowhood and morbidity. In addition, our study sheds light on social connectedness, widowhood, and health. Limitations of many previous studies examining short-term effects of widowhood include cross-sectional data, lack of data about the specific timing of marital status transitions, and little information about individual characteristics. This study addresses these limitations by using a nationally representative longitudinal survey of older people in the United States. The survey includes precise timing information about the transition to widowhood, and permits controls for an extensive set of individual characteristics that have been found to be associated with health and use of health care services.

METHODS

Data

Data are from the 1984, 1986, 1988, and 1990 waves of the Longitudinal Study of Aging (LSOA). The LSOA provides nationally representative measures of the health status of older individuals, and of their use of health care resources over time. The baseline 1984 survey was administered to 7,527 non-institutionalized individuals age 70 or older. Those who later entered nursing homes were included in the follow-up interviews. Kovar, Fitti, and Chyba (1992) provide LSOA details. This study is restricted to 1,460 LSOA women who were married at the time of the baseline survey. A match to Medicare records obtained hospitalization information. Hospitalization records span November 29, 1983, through December 31, 1991. Although the youngest age in the LSOA surveys was 70, some women were still age 69 at the time of a first hospitalization in the available data. Thus, the youngest age represented in the data is age 69. Hospitalization information is unavailable in Medicare records for health maintenance organization (HMO) enrollees among LSOA respondents. Also, identifying information was not obtained from some respondents, or did not match Medicare files (Kovar et al., 1992). The final sample represents 1,138 women for whom the Medicare file match was successful. Weighted analysis was conducted, to account for both the sampling probabilities of the LSOA and the probability of a successful Medicare file match. The later adjustment was made to LSOA weights using procedures described by Aykan, Freedman, and Martin (1999), and accounts for differential probabilities of a successful Medicare file match associated with all baseline variables in the multivariate model.

Conceptual Model Development

The conceptual model of hospitalization risk is based on Andersen's (1989) behavioral model of health service use, extended to include older individuals by Wolinsky and Johnson (1991). The model hypothesizes that health service use is a function of characteristics that predispose people to use services, enable their use, or create a need for their use. Given our focus on social connectedness, social contacts are included in a separate category.

Predisposing Factors are characteristics of individuals that affect their propensity to use health services, and are largely independent of their initial health care needs. Being widowed in the past two years is included as a predisposing factor. Based on previous research that has found the transition to widowhood is associated with a higher risk of death and poorer health (Feldman et al., 2000; Goldman et al., 1995), women who are recently widowed should have a greater risk of hospitalization. Previous research has not examined mechanisms that would produce this increased risk. Stress has been linked to increased disease risk for older individuals (Wylkle, Kahana, & Kowal, 1992), and may be one such mechanism. Recently widowed women may also take on less healthy lifestyles, or may be less pro-active in health care decision-making (Umberson, 1992). These problems may be aggravated by the fact that recently widowed women are more likely to experience depression (Mendes de Leon et al., 1994). However, some evidence exists that women who have been widowed for longer periods may overcome any greater health risks associated with an initial bereavement period (Byles et al., 1999). Thus, we expect that women who have been widowed for longer periods should have a hospitalization risk that differs little from that of women whose husbands remain alive. Race and ethnicity are included as a predisposing factor. A large body of research indicates that race and ethnicity are associated with individuals' predispositions to use health care, involving trust in individual providers and health care institutions (Institute of Medicine, 2002). Increasing age should be positively associated with hospitalization risk. The home is an important source of wealth, and may provide potential heirs with an incentive to prevent erosion of the home's value by minimizing health care costs (Greene & Ondrich, 1990). This suggests that potential heirs would generally look more carefully after the health and well-being of homeowners. Thus, home ownership should be associated with reduced hospitalization risk. A nursing home stay may signal a predisposition to use health services, and may therefore be associated with a higher risk of hospitalization.

Enabling Factors include the ability to comply with prescribed health regimens, and to influence physician discretion in the hospitalization decision. Knowledge of healthy lifestyles and preventive health care services should be greater for the more highly educated. Thus, educational attainment should be negatively associated with hospitalization risk. Another included socioeconomic indicator is income, which should be negatively associated with hospitalization risk. Children, particularly daughters, are likely to provide health-related information and care. Thus, having daughters should be associated with reduced hospitalization risk. Having daughters was selected for use in this study because older women usually prefer to receive care from daughters, rather than from sons (Lee, Dwyer, & Coward, 1993).

Although associated with need, the number of annual physician office visits is included as a measure of preventive care and physician continuity; a greater number of physician visits should be associated with reduced hospitalization risk. Community service use is included as an indicator of knowledge about services that maintain health and well-being, and willingness to use them. From this perspective, greater service use should be associated with a lower risk of hospitalization. Service use may also indicate greater need, and, therefore, greater hospitalization risk. Having private insurance should be positively associated with access to primary and preventive health services, and, therefore, with a lower hospitalization risk. Rural residents and residents of Core Standard Metropolitan Statistical Areas (SMSAs), highly urbanized areas at the center of SMSAs, are more likely to live in primary care physician shortage areas (U.S. Physician Payment Review Commission, 1992). They should therefore be more likely to have conditions that become severe enough to warrant hospitalization. Region of residence is associated with variation in care levels, specialist supply, and thresholds of disease severity at which hospitalization is considered necessary (Wennberg, Fisher, & Skinner, 2002), and is included in the models to control for these health system characteristics.

Need Factors are characteristics of individuals associated with health, disease, and functional status. Self-rated health is a strong predictor of morbidity and hospital use independent of other physiological, behavioral, and psychosocial risk factors (Wolinsky, Culler, Callahan, & Johnson, 1994). Comorbidities included are: heart disease, hypertension, obesity, Alzheimer's Disease and other dementias, arthritis, and diabetes. Comorbidities should be associated with greater need, and thus should be associated with a higher risk of hospitalization. Disability, measured by impairments in ADLs, often explains much of the variance in health care use (Auchincloss, Van Nostrand, & Ronsaville, 2001). Measured ADLs are: bathing or showering, dressing, eating, getting in and out of bed or chairs, walking, getting outside, and using the toilet. The number of previous hospitalizations also indicates need; a greater number should be associated with a higher risk of hospitalization. Time since a previous discharge, on the other hand, should be negatively associated with the admission risk.

Social Contacts. In addition to these predisposing, enabling, and need characteristics, one of our models estimates effects of social contacts. Although a number of social contact measures are available in the LSOA, most are likely to be related to the outcome variable. For example, married women who do not go to the movies or sporting events, or do volunteer work or attend church, may be restricted to the home by health conditions or the health needs of their spouses. We selected two measures of social contact that are less likely to be related to widowhood and hospitalization, having spoken by telephone to a friend or neighbor in the two weeks prior to the baseline interview, or having spoken by telephone to a relative in the same period. Of women who experience a husband's death during the study and report not having telephoned in either of these categories at baseline, only five did not own a telephone, and all but two reported either that they could use a telephone themselves, or that they had help to use one when needed.

Variable Coding

Dependent Variable. The dependent variable indicates whether a hospitalization for any reason occurred during a given 30-day period.

Fixed Variables from the Baseline Interview. A dichotomous variable, Minority Status, indicates whether the respondent was identified by the LSOA as either black, Hispanic, or Aleut, Eskimo, or American Indian. Education in Years is a fixed continuous covariate indicating 0-18 years of education. Our income measure assigns each individual to one of nine income ranges. A dummy variable indicates whether each woman has at least one living daughter. Rural residence is assigned for women living in counties with fewer than 20,000 people. Core SMSA residence identifies women residing in counties with a population of at least one million in 1980 containing the primary central city of the SMSA. Region of residence was also measured at baseline; the omitted category for region is South. Baseline measures should adequately represent rural or SMSA residence, as well as region, throughout the longitudinal study. Only two women made any interstate move during the study period; only thirteen others made an intercounty move. A continuous variable counts community services used at baseline (0-8). Self-rated fair or poor health was included in the models separately, with good to excellent health the omitted category. A dummy variable indicates whether the respondent had a telephone conversation with a friend/neighbor in the two weeks prior to the baseline interview. An analogous variable indicates whether she had a conversation with a relative.

Time Varying Interview Variables. Values of some time varying variables in the models are determined by interviews. Their values from the first wave are assigned from the beginning of the data record through the midpoint of the interval between the first and second interviews. Values from the second interview are assigned from this point through the midpoint between the second and third interviews. Values from later waves are assigned analogously. Interview dates are identified separately for each individual, as are the midpoints. Interview variables are home ownership, nursing home residence, and having private insurance. Because precise dates of nursing home entry and exit are not known in the LSOA, this variable indicates that a woman has one or more nursing home stays during the period associated with each interview. The ADL variable is a count of activities in which the woman is considered to be disabled. A respondent is considered to be disabled in an ADL if she indicated she had "a lot" of difficulty with the activity, or was unable to perform it.

Time Varying Variables from Interviews and Medicare Files. Interviews asked the number of physician office visits in the previous year. The median was four; a physician use dummy variable identifies those with four or more in the period associated with each interview. Several sources provide comorbidity information, including self-reports at baseline, reports in each survey wave of diseases causing impairments, and hospital diagnoses. When a chronic condition is self-reported or appears as a hospital diagnosis, it is assigned to the six prior months, and through the remainder of the study period. Comorbidities are modeled as secondary conditions that may contribute to hospitalization risk, but that are not the primary hospitalization cause, using a method developed and validated by Elixhauser, Steiner, Harris, and Coffey (1998). Between baseline and the first discharge, and between any two discharges, current comorbidity values are separately compared to the primary diagnosis of the next (or current) hospitalization. Where they match, or might be causally related, the comorbidity is coded zero through the next (or current) hospitalization. Obesity is assigned from hospital diagnoses, and when body mass index (BMI), calculated from baseline height and weight, exceeds 32.3. The comorbidity measure entered in the models is a count of the number of existing comorbidities (0-6) for each measured interval at risk.

Time Varying Variables Known to the Day. For women with a hospitalization, birth date is known to the day. For others, birth date is known to the month, and is assigned to the 15th day of that month. Age is entered in the model as age in years minus 69. Thus, the constant refers to age 69. The data enable marital status assignment to the day. However, the dates of marital status change are obtained during interviews, and women who die or attrit cannot thereafter provide this retrospective information. To avoid bias in our estimates of widowhood effects introduced by death or attrition and this subsequent information loss (Koreman et al., 1997), observations with no later interview information are removed from the risk set as of the day following the final completed interview. For each day of the study, a dummy variable indicates whether each woman was widowed within the previous two years, measured to the day. All duration measures are also assigned to the day. The number of previous hospitalizations and days since a previous discharge are set to zero at baseline. Days since a previous discharge are entered in the model divided by 90. Thus, the covariate indicates the change in the hazard associated with each additional 90-day period.

The Hazard Models

The approach uses discrete-time hazard modeling, in which the outcome is modeled as a repeatable event. The hazard expresses the probability that a woman will experience a hospitalization in a 30-day period, given that she is at risk of a hospitalization at that time. All women who are not hospitalized are at risk of a hospitalization. The hospital admission hazard represents 76,678 person intervals.

We estimate three models. The first is designed to identify the comparison group for the remaining models. Based on theory and previous research (Byles et al., 1999; Feldman et al., 2000), we hypothesize that illness levels among women who have been widowed for more than two years should not differ importantly from illness levels among women whose husbands remain alive. To test this hypothesis, we estimate the hazard of hospitalization with the risk set restricted to women who are widowed more than two years, together with those still married. Being widowed more than two years is included in this model as the independent variable of interest. In addition to this covariate, the model includes all controls of our primary analysis.

The primary analysis identifies whether women who have been widowed in the two previous years have a different hospitalization risk than other women who were married at the baseline interview. For this primary model of our analysis, the covariate of interest identifies whether the respondent at any given person-interval was widowed in the two previous years. The third model is designed to test the hypothesis that social connectedness at baseline protects a woman who is later widowed from deteriorating health during the two-year period of initial bereavement. This model adds to the primary analysis model covariates for speaking by telephone to a friend/neighbor, or to a relative. Also added are terms for the interactions of these social contact measures with the covariate indicating whether a given 30-day interval is within the two-year bereavement period.

Estimating discrete-time hazard models involves repeated measures on individuals. A separate observation is created for each 30-day interval for each woman. At each observation, the outcome variable takes the value 1 or 0, indicating that a hospitalization did or did not occur during that interval. Thus, the analytic dataset includes multiple observations for each woman, one for each 30-day period of the study that she remained alive. Logistic regression is applied to this data to estimate the hospitalization hazard. The multiple observations created for the analysis violate a well known assumption of logistic analysis, which is that the observations studied are not importantly correlated, a phenomenon commonly called data dependence. It is also well known that estimates from discrete-time hazard models using logistic regression can be subject to considerable bias resulting from unmeasured heterogeneity. Previous research on use of health services by older individuals using similar modeling strategies, primarily to study the hazard of nursing home use, have generally been conducted with the implicit assumption that all notable sources of heterogeneity have been accounted for in the model specification (Garber & MaCurdy, 1990; Greene & Ondrich, 1990; Laditka, 1998). Where the models fully capture all important variables that contribute to the process under study, all heterogeneity is measured, and any bias in the estimates is eliminated. It is unlikely that most model specifications will successfully eliminate all influential sources of unmeasured heterogeneity, however, even if time-dependence and other important sources of variation are included in the model. Individuals and their environments differ greatly, and a given set of measured covariates may not capture all variation among them.

We investigated the influence of data dependence on our estimates, along with that of other sources of unmeasured heterogeneity, using a random effect specification estimated with MLwiN software. The variance estimate was small and not statistically significant, which suggests that our models are not notably biased by these characteristics. The random effect was therefore not retained in the model. Nonetheless, applying standard logistic analysis to the multiple observations on individual women in our data might produce artificially low standard errors, which could cause misleading estimates of statistical significance. We therefore estimated robust standard errors, which account for this characteristic of the data, using the SAS GENMOD procedure.

RESULTS

Descriptive statistics are shown in Table 1. Most of the women in the sample are white (about 92%), and most own their own homes (82%). The average baseline age of women in the sample is 75.1 years, and

TABLE 1. Baseline Sample Descriptive Measures, Women Married at Baseline (n = 1,138), 1984-1990 Longitudinal Study of Aging

	Mean	(SD)
Predisposing Characteristics		
Minority Status	0.083	(0.275)
Age in Years	75.132	(4.304)
Owns Home	0.820	(0.384)
Nursing Home Stay	0.001	(0.030)
Enabling Characteristics		
Education in Years	10.564	(3.152)
Family Income Category[a]	3.571	(1.943)
Has Living Daughters	0.629	(0.483)
Physician Visits ≥ 4 in Previous 12 Months	0.455	(0.498)
Number of Community Services Used (0-8)	0.349	(0.778)
Has Private Insurance	0.813	(0.390)
Lives in a Core SMSA County	0.221	(0.415)
Lives in a Rural County	0.213	(0.409)
Region, Northeast	0.216	(0.412)
Region, North Central	0.273	(0.446)
Region, West	0.175	(0.380)
Need Characteristics		
Fair Self-Rated Health at Baseline	0.220	(0.414)
Poor Self-Rated Health at Baseline	0.100	(0.300)
Comorbidity Index (0-6)[b]	1.379	(0.985)
Number of ADL Impairments (0-7)	0.258	(0.896)
Social Contacts		
Spoke to Friend/Neighbor by Telephone	0.914	(0.281)
Spoke to Relative by Telephone	0.877	(0.329)
Women Ever in Two-Year Bereavement Period, 1984-1990, n	302	

[a]Income Category 3: $10,000 - $14,999; income category 4: $15,000-$19,999.
[b]Comorbidity Index is the sum of indicator variables for baseline measures of heart disease, hypertension, diabetes, obesity, Alzheimer's Disease and other dementias, and arthritis.

their average educational attainment is 10.5 years. The majority of women have at least one living daughter (63%) and private insurance in addition to Medicare (81%). About 33% of women in the sample rated their health as either fair or poor at baseline. Most women telephoned a friend/neighbor (91%) or relative (88%) in the two-week period prior to their baseline interviews. Both a friend/neighbor contact and relative contact were made by 82.5% of respondents (not shown). Of the 1,138 women in our analytical sample, 302 (27%) were widowed during the study period.

The hazard model designed to identify whether women widowed more than two years have a different hospitalization risk from those whose husbands remain alive is not shown. The odds ratio on the covariate identifying those widowed more than two years is 1.0056 ($p = 0.0121$). Although statistically significant, the small magnitude of this estimate suggests no meaningful difference in hospitalization risk between women in these two groups. Given this finding, the comparison group for the remaining models includes all women married at baseline who are not within a two-year period of initial bereavement, including both those whose husbands remain alive and those widowed more than two years.

The remaining hazard model results are reported in Table 2. The data columns at the left of the Table show our primary model, which identifies whether women in a two-year period of initial bereavement have a greater risk of hospitalization than all other women. The model depicted at the right of Table 2 adds covariates associated with social contacts. For both models, Table 2 shows coefficients and standard errors, standard levels of statistical significance, odds ratio point estimates, and the 95% confidence interval (CI) for the odds ratios. For continuous variables, the reported odds ratio point estimate and 95% CI is $100(e^{\beta}-1)$, the percent change in the odds for each 1-unit increase in the covariate value. Given the focus of this study on health effects of recent widowhood and the mitigating role of social connectedness, we limit our discussion to these characteristics.

In the primary model of the analysis, controlling for other predisposing factors and for enabling and need characteristics, the odds of hospitalization for a recently widowed woman are nearly 40% greater than the odds for all other women who were married at baseline (odds ratio 1.38, 95% CI 1.12~1.69, $p < 0.01$). In the second model, which includes main effects and interaction terms for social contacts, the main effect estimate for being Within Two-Year Bereavement Period indicates that the odds of a recently widowed woman with neither social contact being

TABLE 2. 30-Day Hazard of Hospital Admission, Women Married at Baseline (n = 1,138), 1984-1990 Longitudinal Study of Aging

			Odds Ratio	95% CI				Odds Ratio	95% CI	
	b	(SE)		LB	UB	b	(SE)		LB	UB
Predisposing Characteristics										
Within Two-Year Bereavement Period	0.3199	(0.1040)**	1.38	1.12	1.69	1.2598	(0.2710)***	3.52	2.07	5.99
Minority Status[a]	-0.0110	(0.0706)	0.99	0.86	1.14	-0.0012	(0.0687)	1.00	0.87	1.14
Age in Years[a]	0.0261	(0.0039)***	2.64	1.87	3.43	0.0255	(0.0039)***	2.58	1.80	3.37
Owns Home	0.1000	(0.0508)*	1.11	1.00	1.22	0.1000	(0.0507)*	1.11	1.00	1.22
Nursing Home Stay	-0.2241	(0.1088)*	0.80	0.65	0.99	-0.2001	(0.1119)+	0.82	0.66	1.02
Enabling Characteristics										
Education in Years[a]	-0.0053	(0.0059)	-0.53	-1.68	0.64	-0.0062	(0.0061)	-0.62	-1.79	0.56
Family Income Category (0-8)[a]	0.0221	(0.0092)*	2.23	0.40	4.10	0.0233	(0.0095)*	2.36	0.47	4.27
Has Living Daughters	-0.0131	(0.0334)	0.99	0.92	1.05	-0.0071	(0.0347)	0.99	0.93	1.06
Physician Visits ≥ 4 in Previous 12 Months	0.0271	(0.0502)	1.03	0.93	1.13	0.0354	(0.0508)	1.04	0.94	1.14
Number of Community Services Used (0-8)[a]	0.0123	(0.0224)	1.24	-3.11	5.79	0.0165	(0.0224)	1.66	-2.71	6.24
Has Private Insurance	-0.0355	(0.0420)	0.97	0.89	1.05	-0.0445	(0.0431)	0.96	0.88	1.04
Lives in a Core SMSA County	-0.0061	(0.0450)	0.99	0.91	1.09	-0.0012	(0.0454)	1.00	0.91	1.09
Lives in a Rural County	0.0199	(0.0385)	1.02	0.95	1.10	0.0199	(0.0392)	1.02	0.94	1.10
Region, Northeast	-0.0291	(0.0490)	0.97	0.88	1.07	-0.0305	(0.0488)	0.97	0.88	1.07
Region, North Central	-0.0044	(0.0404)	1.00	0.92	1.08	-0.0055	(0.0409)	0.99	0.92	1.08
Region, West	-0.0090	(0.0468)	0.99	0.90	1.09	-0.0071	(0.0471)	0.99	0.91	1.09
Need Characteristics										
Fair Self-Rated Health at Baseline	0.0474	(0.0360)	1.05	0.98	1.13	0.0553	(0.0369)	1.06	0.98	1.14
Poor Self-Rated Health at Baseline	-0.0555	(0.0701)	0.95	0.82	1.09	-0.0537	(0.0720)	0.95	0.82	1.09
Comorbidity Index (0-6)[a]	0.0551	(0.0175)**	5.66	2.10	9.36	0.0499	(0.0177)**	5.12	1.53	8.83
Number of ADL Impairments (0-7)[a]	-0.0081	(0.0194)	-0.81	-4.51	3.05	-0.0093	(0.0202)	-0.93	-4.77	3.09
Number of Previous Hospitalizations[a]	0.2329	(0.0152)***	26.23	22.51	30.06	0.2349	(0.0154)***	26.48	22.70	30.37
Days Since Last Discharge/90[a]	-0.3390	(0.0295)***	-28.75	-32.76	-24.51	-0.3380	(0.0295)***	-28.68	-32.68	-24.44
Social Contacts										
Spoke to Friend/Neighbor by Telephone						0.0682	(0.0710)	1.07	0.93	1.23
Spoke to Relative by Telephone						0.0367	(0.0856)	1.04	0.88	1.23
Phoned Friend × Bereavement Period						-0.4717	(0.2252)*	0.62	0.40	0.97
Phoned Relative × Bereavement Period						-0.5765	(0.2704)*	0.56	0.33	0.95
Constant	-6.3797	(0.2495)***				-6.4692	(0.2594)***			
-2 x Log Likelihood	17,306					17,302				

[a] Reported for continuous variables, including 95% Confidence Interval (CI), is $100(e^{\beta}-1)$, the percent change in the risk for each 1-unit increase in the covariate value.

+ $p < 0.1$, * $p < 0.05$, ** $p < 0.01$, *** $p < 0.001$

hospitalized are over 3.5 times greater than the odds of hospitalization for other women in the sample (odds ratio 3.52, 95% CI 2.07~5.99, $p < 0.001$). The interaction effects are both statistically significant. The odds of hospitalization for a woman in the initial bereavement period who spoke to a friend/neighbor in the two weeks prior to the baseline interview are given by: $e^{-6.4692} \times e^{1.2598} \times e^{0.0682} \times e^{-0.4717} = 0.00365$, holding all other model covariates at their zero or reserved category levels. The corresponding odds for a woman in the initial bereavement period who did *not* speak to a friend/neighbor are given by: $e^{-6.4692} \times e^{1.2598} = 0.005464$. Thus, the odds ratio for hospitalization during the initial bereavement period, comparing women having a friend/neighbor contact with those who did not, is: $0.00365/0.005464 = 0.67$ (see DeMaris, 1992, for a description of such calculations). So the odds of a recently widowed woman with this form of social contact having such a hospitalization are about 33% lower than the odds for a recently widowed woman without this social contact. The corresponding odds ratio comparing those who had contacts with relatives to those who did not is 0.58. Thus, the odds of hospitalization during the initial bereavement period for a woman with this form of social contact are over 40% lower than the odds of hospitalization for a recently widowed woman without this contact.

Finally, we compared the types of hospitalizations experienced by women who were recently widowed and those who were not. The results, summarized by Major Diagnosis Categories (MDCs), are shown in Table 3. There were a total of 1,430 hospitalizations included in our analysis, 135 experienced by women during the two-year period of initial bereavement, and 1,295 by women who were not recently widowed. As displayed in Table 3, the most common MDCs were the same for both groups of women: (1) circulatory related conditions (e.g., heart failure, angina, cardiac arrhythmias); (2) musculoskeletal and connective tissue conditions (e.g., back related problems, hip procedures); and (3) digestive disorders (e.g., gastrointestinal obstruction). Overall, the analysis of hospitalization types showed that the reasons for hospitalization were similar for these groups and appeared to be randomly distributed for women who were recently widowed. There were no highly discretionary, elective procedures for women in either group. Restricting analysis to the 11 data rows of Table 3 having at least four hospitalizations in the column representing the two-year bereavement period, results of the Cochran-Mantel-Haenszel test of general association (Stokes, Davis, & Koch, 1995) suggest that the distribution of hospitalizations among these diagnosis categories does not differ between

TABLE 3. Major Diagnostic Categories (MDCs) for Hospitalizations in Two-Year Bereavement Period and All Other Hospitalizations, Women Married at Baseline (n = 1,138), 1984-1990 Longitudinal Study of Aging

MDC Code	MDC Category	Hospitalizations Not During Two-Year Bereavement		Hospitalizations During Two-Year Bereavement	
		N	%	N	%
5	Diseases & Disorders Of The Circulatory System	307	23.71	37	27.41
8	Diseases & Disorders Of The Musculoskeletal System & Connective Tissues	222	17.14	21	15.56
6	Diseases & Disorders Of The Digestive System	183	14.13	16	11.85
4	Diseases & Disorders Of The Respiratory System	113	8.73	6	4.44
1	Diseases & Disorders Of The Nervous System	91	7.03	14	10.37
10	Endocrine, Nutritional & Metabolic Diseases & Disorders	49	3.78	8	5.93
7	Diseases & Disorders Of The Hepatobiliary System & Pancreas	48	3.71	4	2.96
13	Diseases & Disorders Of The Female Reproductive System	43	3.32	0	0
9	Diseases & Disorders Of The Skin, Subcutaneous Tissue & Breast	42	3.24	4	2.96
11	Diseases & Disorders Of The Kidney & Urinary Tract	35	2.70	6	4.44
2	Diseases & Disorders Of The Eye	30	2.32	5	3.7
17	Myeloproliferative Diseases & Disorders, Poorly Differentiated	28	2.16	0	0
3	Diseases & Disorders Of The Ear, Nose, Mouth & Throat	24	1.85	0	0
19	Mental Diseases & Disorders	19	1.47	6	4.44
24	Multiple Significant Trauma	15	1.16	2	1.48
21	Injuries, Poisonings & Toxic Effects Of Drugs	13	1.00	1	0.74
18	Infectious & Parasitic Diseases, Systemic Or Unspecified Sites	10	0.77	2	1.48
16	Diseases & Disorders Of Blood, Blood Forming Organs, Immunological	9	0.69	1	0.74
23	Factors Influencing Health Status & Other Contacts With Health Services	6	0.46	1	0.74
20	Alcohol/Drug Use & Alcohol/Drug Induced Organic Mental Disorders	2	0.15	1	0.74
	Missing Values And Illegal Codes	6	0.46	0	0
	Total Hospitalizations	1295		135	

the two groups of women ($\chi^2 = 14.62$, df = 10, p = .15). Analyses incorporating the remaining diagnoses provide unreliable chi-square statistics, due to the proportion of cells with counts less than five, and are not reported.

DISCUSSION AND POLICY IMPLICATIONS

The number of older people is growing rapidly. Their growing number also brings an increase in the number of women who experience a husband's death. Yet surprisingly little research has examined the relationship between bereavement and health. Most related research has focused on the association between recent widowhood and mortality. Our study explored the relationship between bereavement and health, using hospitalization as a health status indicator.

Our primary finding is that recently widowed women have nearly 40% higher risk of hospitalization than women not recently widowed. We also found that the hospitalization risk for women who have been widowed for more than two years does not differ importantly from that of women whose husbands remain alive. These findings are consistent with research that has found recently widowed women have a higher mortality risk than women not recently widowed (e.g., Lillard & Waite, 1995). They are also consistent with the few studies that have examined the association between recent widowhood and morbidity with cross-sectional analyses (e.g., Byles et al., 1999). We build on the few prior studies of bereavement and morbidity by using a nationally representative sample of older women studied longitudinally. Our data update marital status and hospitalization information for each day of the study, and account for losses due to attrition or death (Korenman et al., 1997). Our models include controls for predisposing, enabling, and need characteristics that have previously been found to be associated with health and hospitalization (Andersen, 1989; Wolinsky & Johnson, 1991).

Our study also examined the mediating effect of social connectedness on health among older women who were recently widowed. We found that, among recent widows, the socially isolated have a substantially higher risk of hospitalization than do women having contacts with family or friends/neighbors. Our results for social connectedness are consistent with research on the association between widowhood and mortality (e.g., Goldman et al., 1995), and shed new light on the role of social connectedness and health among recently widowed older women. An advantage of the social contact indicators we used, talking by telephone with family or friends/neighbors, is that these measures may be less closely related to health and hospitalization than other common measures of social connectedness. Aside from the most severely physically impaired and those with extreme cognitive impairment, most women can participate in the social activity measured in this study. The measure is also unlikely to be importantly biased by a husband's ability to participate in social activities outside the home.

As Goldman et al. (1995) note, it would be preferable to have social contact information collected at follow-up interviews as well as at baseline. The baseline measure may be biased to the extent that women substantially change their social connectedness, either in the period preceding a husband's death, or in the period that follows. Utz, Carr, Nesse, and Wortman (2002) examined how social participation changes in response to widowhood at older ages. They found that informal participation, such as contact with family and friends, increases following a husband's death. However, they also found support for the continuity theory, that prior social contacts are the strongest predictor of social participation after widowhood.

The data and method used for our analysis permitted an exploration of a rarely studied topic and can be expected to produce reasonably robust results. Nonetheless, the data imposed some limitations. The level of generalization of the income ranges reported by the LSOA, together with limited ability to accurately identify changing family size throughout the study period, did not permit an adjustment to income for household scale economies. The comorbidity scale, a summed index of six comorbidity measures, should have reasonable reliability. Self-reported comorbidities in our data are for the most part for common conditions with relatively simple diagnoses. Self-reports of such conditions have been found to be reasonably reliable (Baker, Stabile, & Deri, 2001), and our comorbidity definitions are augmented with provider diagnoses reported from hospitalizations. Summing these comorbidities in a scale is consistent with previous research (Blustein, Hanson, & Shea, 1998). However, such scales assume that each comorbidity contributes equally to the process under study. There is little theoretical justification to support this assumption (Elixhauser et al., 1998). Days Since Last Discharge are unmeasured at baseline. A common approach addressed this, assigning zero days at baseline and including age as a covariate (Allison, 1995). If the number of deaths among recently widowed women were substantial, the results could be biased by selection effects. In this case, those who remain alive to later widowhood might generally have better health, in dimensions not measured by our multivariate models, than the women who die during the initial bereavement period. However, there were few deaths among widowed women during the study period. Six women died during the two-year period of initial bereavement. Another seven women died more than two years after their husbands' deaths.

This study has several implications for social policy, for older women, and for their families and caregivers. From a policy perspective, our finding that the health status of recently widowed women is substantially worse than that of married women, or of women who were widowed in the more distant past, highlights the need to focus resources toward women in this high risk group. Community-based organizations, such as senior day centers, could offer special support groups for women who are recently widowed. Organizations such as the local office for aging might provide routine screenings and emphasize the role of preventive care targeted particularly for recently widowed older individuals. The recent reauthorization of the Older Americans Act provides states with additional funding to provide support and guidance for caregivers. Community caregiver support centers, for example, might offer support groups for families and caregivers to highlight the special needs of recently widowed women. When designing eldercare training, employers could emphasize health risks for those who are recently widowed. There are also implications for practitioners. Primary care physicians, geriatric nurse practitioners, and social workers should be made aware that recent widowhood is an important risk factor for declining health and hospitalization. Given high costs of hospitalization and the substantially increased hospitalization risk faced by recent widows, such initiatives are likely to be cost efficient. There are also implications for families and friends of recently widowed women. Our findings that social connectedness can greatly mitigate the adverse health effects of widowhood highlight the importance for family and friends of maintaining regular contact with a recently widowed woman.

Additional research is needed to explore the needs of recently widowed older women and men. Our analysis suggests that the increased risk of poor health and hospitalization in the initial period of bereavement is temporary. Women who were widowed more than two years faced no notably different hospitalization risk than those whose husbands remained alive. Nonetheless, a woman's substantially increased risk of hospitalization during the two years following a husband's death deserves attention. Risks of hospitalization for older individuals include adverse drug events, falls, nosocomial infections, pressure sores, surgical and postoperative complications, functional decline, delirium, and substandard or negligent care (Creditor, 1993). These risks can often result in loss of independence following discharge, with additional costs of formal or informal care. Hospitalization of older people also has great economic costs, both for individuals and for Medicare. The findings of our study suggest that providers and policy makers should consider ways to support recently widowed women. One useful starting point might be for us all to offer more support to older recently widowed women among our friends and families.

REFERENCES

Allison, P.D. (1995). Survival analysis using the SAS system: A practical guide. Cary, NC: SAS Institute, Inc.

Andersen, R.M. (1989). A behavioral model of families' use of health services. Chicago: Center for Administration Studies.

Anson, O. (1989). Marital status and women's health revisited: The importance of a proximate adult. *Journal of Marriage and the Family, 51*, 185-202.

Antonucci, T.C., & Akiyama, H. (1987). An examination of sex differences in social support among older men and women. *Sex Roles, 17*, 737-749.

Auchincloss, A.H., Van Nostrand, J.F., & Ronsaville, D. (2001). Access to health care for older persons in the United States: Personal, structural, and neighborhood characteristics. *Journal of Aging and Health, 13*, 329-354.

Aykan, H., Freedman, V.A., & Martin, L.G. (1999). *Re-weighting the Second Supplement on Aging to the 1994 National Health Interview Survey for trend analyses.* RAND Labor and Population Program Working Paper No. 99-05. (DRU-2006) Santa Monica, CA: RAND.

Baker, M., Stabile, M., & Deri, C. (2001). What do self-reported, objective, measures of health measure? National Bureau of Economic Research (NBER) Working Paper No. W8419.

Blustein, J., Hanson, K., & Shea, S. (1998). Preventable hospitalizations and socioeconomic status. *Health Affairs 17*, 177-189.

Bound, J., Duncon, G.J., Laren, D.S., & Oleinick, L. (1991). Poverty dynamics in widowhood. *Journal of Gerontology: Social Sciences, 46*, S115-S124.

Burkhauser, R.V., & Smeeding, T.M. (1994). *Social Security reform: A budget neutral approach to reducing older women's disproportionate risk of poverty.* Policy Brief Series. Center for Policy Research, Maxwell School. Syracuse, NY: Syracuse University.

Byles, J., Feldman, S., & Mishra, G. (1999). For richer, for poorer, in sickness and in health: Older widowed women's health, relationships and financial security. *Women & Health, 29*, 15-29.

Creditor, M.C. (1993). Hazards of hospitalization of the elderly. *Annals of Internal Medicine, 118*, 220-223.

DeMaris, A. (1992). *Logit modeling: Practical applications.* Newbury Park, CA: Sage.

Elixhauser, A., Steiner C., Harris, R., & Coffey, R.M. (1998). Comorbidity measures for use with administrative data. *Medical Care, 35*, 8-27.

Feldman, S., Byles, J.E., & Beaumont, R. (2000). 'Is anybody listening?' The experiences of widowhood for older Australian women. *Journal of Women & Aging, 12,* 155-176.

Garber, A.M., & MaCurdy, T. (1990). Predicting nursing home utilization among the high-risk elderly. In D.A. Wise (Ed.), *Issues in the Economics of Aging* (pp. 173-204). Chicago, IL: University of Chicago Press.

Goldman, N., Korenman, S., & Weinstein, R. (1995). Marital status and health among the elderly. *Social Science and Medicine, 40,* 1717-1730.

Greene, V.L., & Ondrich, J.I. (1990). Risk factors for nursing home admissions and exits: A discrete-time hazard function approach. *Journal of Gerontology: Social Sciences, 45,* S250-S258.

Hu, K., & Goldman, N. (1990). Mortality differentials by marital status: An international comparison. *Demography, 27,* 233-250.

Institute of Medicine. (2002). *Unequal treatment: Confronting racial and ethnic disparities in health care.* Washington, D.C.: National Academy Press. Available at: <://www4.nationalacademies.org/>. Accessed March 23, 2002.

Kinsella, K. (2000). Demographic dimensions of global aging. *Journal of Family Issues, 21,* 541-558.

Kirschling, J.M., & McBride, A.B. (1989). Effects of age and sex on the experience of widowhood. *Western Journal of Nursing Research, 11,* 207-218.

Korenman, S., Goldman, N., & Fu, H. (1997). Misclassification bias in estimates of bereavement effects. *American Journal of Epidemiology, 145,* 995-1001.

Kovar, M.G., Fitti, J.E., & Chyba, M.M. (1992). *The Longitudinal Study of Aging: 1984-1990.* Vital Health Statistics (28, no. 1), Hyattsville, MD, National Center for Health Statistics.

Kravdal, Ø. (2001). The impact of marital status on cancer survival. *Social Science and Medicine, 52,* 357-368.

Laditka, S.B. (1998). Modeling lifetime nursing home use under assumptions of better health. *Journal of Gerontology: Social Sciences, 53B,* S177-S187.

Lee, G.R., Dwyer, J.W., & Coward, R.T. (1993). Gender differences in parent care: Demographic factors and same-gender preferences. *Journal of Gerontology: Social Sciences, 48,* S9-S16.

Lillard, L.A., & Waite, L.J. (1995). Til death do us part: Marital disruption and mortality. *American Journal of Sociology, 100,* 1131-1156.

Mendes De Leon, C.F., Kasl, V., & Jacobs, S. (1994). A prospective study of widowhood and changes in symptoms of depression in a community sample of the elderly. *Psychological Medicine, 24,* 613-624.

Porter, E.J. (1995). The life-world of older widows: The context of lived experience. *Journal of Women & Aging, 7,* 31-16.

Stokes, M.E., Davis, C.S., & Koch, G.G. (1995). *Categorical data analysis using the SAS system.* Cary, NC: SAS Institute, Inc.

Umberson, D. (1992). Gender, marital status, and the social control of health behavior. *Social Science and Medicine, 34,* 907-917.

U.S. Physician Payment Review Commission. (1992). *Increasing the availability of health professionals in shortage areas. 1992 Annual Report to Congress.* Washington, DC: Physician Payment Review Commission.

Utz, R.L., Carr, D., Nesse, R., & Wortman, C.B. (2002). The effect of widowhood on older adults' social participation: An evaluation of activity, disengagement, and continuity theories. *The Gerontologist, 42,* 522-533.

Wennberg, J.E., Fisher, E.S., & Skinner, J.S. (2002). Geography and the debate over Medicare reform. *Health Affairs, 13,* W96-W114. Web publication: <www. healthaffairs.org>. Accessed February 15, 2002.

Wolinsky, F.D., Culler, S.D., Callahan, C.M., & Johnson, R.J. (1994). Hospital resource consumption among older adults: A prospective analysis of episodes, length of stay, and charges over a seven-year period. *Journal of Gerontology: Social Sciences, 49,* S240-S252.

Wolinsky, F.D., & Johnson, R.J. (1991). The use of health services by older adults. *Journal of Gerontology: Social Sciences, 46,* S345-S357.

Wylkle, M.L., Kahana, E., & Kowal, J. (Eds.) (1992). *Stress and health among the elderly.* New York: Springer Publishing Company.

Health, Widowhood, and Family Support in the North and South Pacific: A Comparative Study

James W. McNally, PhD

SUMMARY. This paper compares the impacts of health and widowhood on the level of support received by elderly women living in small island communities within the Philippines and Fiji. Using a theoretical perspective of ongoing reciprocal exchange as opposed to altruistic support within household economies, this paper reviews the impacts of disability and economic contributions on the level of support an elderly female receives. It is hypothesized that as the health of the widow declines her access to care will also diminish due to an inability to contribute to the household economies of the extended family. This paper extends existing work on health and family support of widowed females in the developing world by performing a cross-national comparative analysis as well as by explicitly testing the assumptions of altruism that are a central assumption of most models of long-term care in underdeveloped nations. *[Article copies available for a fee from The Haworth Document Delivery Service: 1-800-HAWORTH. E-mail address: <docdelivery@haworthpress. com> Website: <http://www.HaworthPress.com> © 2003 by The Haworth Press, Inc. All rights reserved.]*

Address correspondence to: James W. McNally, National Archive of Computerized Data on Aging, 426 Thompson Street, Ann Arbor MI 48104 (E-mail: jmcnally@umich.edu).

[Haworth co-indexing entry note]: "Health, Widowhood, and Family Support in the North and South Pacific: A Comparative Study." McNally, James W. Co-published simultaneously in *Journal of Women & Aging* (The Haworth Press, Inc.) Vol. 15, No. 2/3, 2003, pp. 29-47; and: *Widows and Divorcees in Later Life: On Their Own Again* (ed: Carol L. Jenkins) The Haworth Press, Inc., 2003, pp. 29-47. Single or multiple copies of this article are available for a fee from The Haworth Document Delivery Service [1-800-HAWORTH, 9:00 a.m. - 5:00 p.m. (EST). E-mail address: docdelivery@haworthpress.com].

10.1300/J074v15n02_03

KEYWORDS. Disability, widows, care, coresidence, Fiji, Philippines

INTRODUCTION

Our understanding of widowhood in the developing world has undergone a transformation over the past decade. While there is little argument that the care of the elderly remains fixed within the family, the quality and the availability of this care can vary dramatically. The perception of the elderly widow as a valued and respected blessing for a family is being redefined as worldwide advances in longevity and health care increase the absolute number of surviving elderly without parallel gains in their economic security in old age. Increasingly, elderly widows are seen as competitors for limited resources within households where they may lack the power to negotiate successfully for necessary resources or levels of care. When other costs within a household receive a higher priority than those of the elderly widow, she may face a reduced quality of life, increased risk of health impairments or other types of unmet need.

As the research literature increasingly shows that non-coresident kin play a minor role in the care and support of the elderly the relationship between the direct availability of family support and unmet need is central to understanding quality of life issues among widows in the developing world (Rasmussen, 1989; Martin, 1990; Panapasa, 2000). This article argues that the care and support of elderly widows in developing nations is tied to direct and immediate access to family and so it examines coresidence as the central mechanism for maintaining support networks for elderly widows. Specifically this paper seeks to identify factors that predict the likelihood that an elderly widow will reside in the home of a child as opposed to other, less optimal household types.

Employing a cross-cultural perspective, the paper examines these differences in residential choice among elderly widows using of data from the island of Palawan in the Philippines and the island Vanua Levu in Fiji. By employing these geographically isolated communities the analysis allows for a focus on the operation of family support networks in small communities, isolated from the support services of larger urban areas. Through this approach, the article seeks to identify normative patterns of residential choice among the elderly in areas where both housing options and family support mechanisms are limited.

BACKGROUND

Early theories of widowhood in the developing world presented a positive interpretation of elderly females joining their children after the death of their spouse and reaping the benefits of her investment in child-bearing. Concepts such as "retirement fertility" were posited as if the rearing of children acted like a caregiving savings account that could be spent down in old age (Nugent, 1985). Researchers such as Cowgill (1972) idealized the status and power of the elderly in the developing world, arguing that as societies developed the elderly became increasingly disenfranchised. Overall, the elderly in the developing world were perceived as being both well off and well cared for so little effort was invested in understanding the aging lifecourse.

The assumption that families in the developing world would continue their traditional role of caring for their aged without external support has only recently come into question, and many governments are now attempting to address the needs of a growing aged population with little or no gerontological infrastructure in place (United Nations, 1999). Lacking adequate retirement programs, pensions and social support networks, the elderly in the developing world remain largely dependent upon the family for care and support in later life. When the care of an elderly widow falls to the family, it is expressed most efficiently in the form of coresidence (DaVanzo and Chan, 1994; Aghajanian, 1985).

While not a perfect solution to the needs of the elderly, coresidence seems the best alternative given available choice in most developing nations. While Martin (1990) has shown that coresidence does not insure either the quality or consistency of care for the elderly, she (Martin, 1989) has also argued that even after allowing for the potential value of non-coresident support, good health and economic independence, coresidence still represents the best insurance for elderly to obtain adequate care and support on an ongoing basis in developing nations. Similarly, while Vlassoff (1990) and Cain (1991) have debated the relative merits of children as a source of support for widows in rural India, both concur on the importance of the extended family to ensure a higher quality of life among elderly females. Even within the extended household, however, many factors can influence the level of power of the elderly and their ability to negotiate for care and support.

Elderly who contribute to household economies, for example, positively influence the quality and level of support they receive. While family altruism may insure some level of care from family members (Cowgill, 1972; Goody, 1996), acts of reciprocity play an ongoing role in maintaining the status and power of the elderly in extended families. Reciprocity in any form helps to reduce stresses associated with the caretaker burden by reaffirming traditional values of kin support and intergenerational responsibility (Dwyer et al., 1994). In general it has been shown repeatedly that economically active elderly, particularly those with property and the control of resources, will have higher status within the household and more power over decisions affecting the household economies (Mutran and Reitzes, 1984; Williams and Domingo, 1993).

In contrast, the presence of disabling impairments decreases the ability of the elderly to contribute to household economies and thus reduces their ability to negotiate for care at the very time they need it most. While the literature on disability and the elderly in the developing world remains limited, a variety of studies across time from Bowen (1964) to more recent work by Rensal and Howard (1997) uniformly show that the disabled face decreased status and power within the household. There is growing evidence that, when care is tied to in-kind exchanges within the household, the quality of care declines as the elderly become impaired and unable to contribute to household economies (Lillard and Willis, 1997; Panapasa, 2002). Research specifically addressing the status of the elderly in the Pacific has shown that the elderly with the highest levels of disability also tend to live in the poorest households and have the least access to support and care (Panapasa and McNally, 1997). More recently, Panapasa (2002) used disability information from the 1996 Census of Fiji to show that disabled elderly were at much higher risk of living alone than the nondisabled and so faced a greater risk of unmet needs. This paper builds on these studies and tests the joint effects of both economic contribution and level of disability among the elderly in two developing nations to see how these factors influence the ability of the elderly to gain access to a household structure that maximizes their opportunities for care and support.

METHODOLOGY

Research Sites

The analysis presented in this paper examines the residential choice patterns of elderly female widows in rural provinces in the Philippines and in Fiji. One study area is Palawan Province located in the North Pacific nation of the Philippines. As the westernmost island in the Philippines, Palawan contains one small urban center with a primarily rural population whose economy depends largely upon subsistence agriculture and small scale fishing enterprises. The other study area is the island of Vanua Levu located in the South Pacific nation of Fiji. Vanua Levu is the second largest island in the Fiji archipelago and consists of two small periurban centers surrounded by a rural population living primarily in small village communities. Like Palawan, the economic activities of indigenous Fijian population in Vanua Levu are predominantly subsistence farming activities and small scaling fishing. While Palawan is more developed in outlook and worldview, severe limitations in resources and economic opportunities negate these differences and the people of both study areas are self-reliant and community oriented.

The two areas selected for this analysis have been chosen because they both share limited access to the larger, urban cores of the Philippines and Fiji. Due to their geographical isolation, these areas are self-reliant and the people subscribe to traditional norms that reinforce values of cooperation and mutual support. Under these conditions it is assumed that if family care is driven by altruistic values rather than economic rationality, then the weakest and most needy elderly should be most likely to be found in extended households where they will have direct access to care and support. If, however, residential choice is based upon patterns of reciprocity then the disabled and unemployed elderly should face a heightened risk of diminished care or even abandonment. As it is assumed that normative pressures on families to conform to community expectations are powerful in these areas, observable patterns of suboptimal care for elderly widows would suggest tacit approval of this behavior on the part of the community.

Data and Methods

The data for the analysis draw from the 1995 Census of the Philippines and the 1996 Census of Fiji. As these data represent 100 percent individual count data, they allow detailed analysis to be performed upon the small number of elderly widows found in small geographical areas such as Palawan and Vanua Levu. The analysis models residential choice structures among all elderly females living in the study areas who are aged 55 and older and reported they were widowed. This represents 6,300 women from Palawan Province, the Philippines and 1,167 women from the island of Vanua Levu, Fiji. Together they provide a pooled analysis population of 7,467 widows. Table 1 summarizes the means and standard deviations for variables to be employed when examining the analysis population.

TABLE 1. Means and Standard Deviations for Variables Used in Residential Choice Model of Elderly Widows: Palawan, Philippines, and Vanua Levu, Fiji, 1995-1996

	Pooled Data		Palawan		Vanua Levu	
Variable Name	Mean	Std Dev	Mean	Std Dev	Mean	Std Dev
Dependent Variable						
Household Type	1.51	0.88	1.44	0.86	1.91	0.88
Lives Alone	0.09	0.29	0.10	0.30	0.04	0.20
Head of a Complex Home	0.47	0.50	0.50	0.50	0.31	0.46
Lives in Home of Child	0.26	0.44	0.25	0.43	0.34	0.47
Lives in Home of Other	0.17	0.38	0.15	0.35	0.31	0.46
Independent Variables						
Age 55 to 64 Years	0.41	0.49	0.41	0.49	0.37	0.48
Age 65 to 74 Years	0.35	0.48	0.35	0.48	0.36	0.48
Age 75 and Older	0.24	0.43	0.24	0.43	0.27	0.44
No Formal Education	0.16	0.37	0.17	0.37	0.12	0.33
Grade School Education	0.69	0.46	0.69	0.46	0.65	0.48
Secondary Education	0.15	0.36	0.14	0.34	0.23	0.42
No Economic Activity	0.57	0.49	0.58	0.49	0.54	0.50
Has Disability	0.11	0.32	0.11	0.31	0.14	0.35
Unemployed and Disabled	0.08	0.28	0.08	0.27	0.12	0.33
Total N	7,467		6,300		1,167	

The dependent variable of the analysis is a measure of the primary household structure in which the elderly respondent resides. This variable consists of a categorical variable with four levels: (1) Elderly widows who live alone, (2) Elderly widows who are the household heads of complex households, (3) Elderly Widows who live in a home where one of their children is the household head, and 4) Elderly widows who live in the home of another individual who is the household head. Prior studies suggest that living in a household controlled by an adult child represents the residential form offering the highest levels of support and care for elderly widows in both the Philippines and in Fiji. Being a household head or living in the household of another individual, while less optimal still remains preferable to living alone. Because widows who live alone lack direct access to the care and support that coresidence can provide, this residential choice is seen as the least desirable household type and will serve as our reference group for the dependent variable in multivariate analysis.

Widows who live alone are a relatively small group, representing only 10 percent of Palawan widows and 4 percent of Fijian widows. In contrast, headship among widows is surprisingly high for both groups with 50 percent of Palawan widows reporting they are the heads of complex households compared to 31 percent of Fijian widows. This trend may be the result of international and internal labor force migration common in both the Philippines and Fiji that drains many rural areas of working-age adult children. Fijian widows are somewhat more likely to reside in the home of a child, with 34 percent of Fijian widows reporting this residential form compared to 25 percent of Palawan widows. Fijian widows are also more likely to reside in the household of others compared to Filipino widows, with 31 percent reporting this residential form compared to only 15 percent of widows in Palawan.

Age represents an important proxy for both morbidity and mortality. The risk of chronic impairment and disability increases with time, as does the need for increased levels of care and supervision as the elderly progress through the aging lifecourse. Under an altruistic system, we would expect to see increasing numbers of widows living with children and with others as they age and become more dependent upon family support networks for care. In contrast, under a reciprocity model we would expect to see a greater risk of living alone among the elderly as they become less able to assist or contribute to household economies. In general, widows in Palawan and Vanau Levu have similar age structures with 41 percent in the young old categories of 55 to 64 years of age, followed by 35 percent in the old age groups between 65 and 74 years of age and 24 percent of the widowed population in the oldest old categories aged 75 and older.

As no income information is available, educational attainment represents a proxy for socioeconomic status in this analysis. Higher levels of education provide greater opportunities to gain economic security, as well as access to information that can help maintain health and autonomy in later life. While low levels of secondary education attainment remain common in both the Philippines and Fiji, most people have had access to at least some basic education. Only about 15 percent of elderly female widows in both Palawan and Fiji report having no formal education, while 65 percent to 69 percent of these women report at least some grade school education. Widows from Palawan report somewhat lower rates of secondary education (14 percent) compared to widows from Fiji (23 percent).

As we lack direct measures of wage income and in-kind contributions for both countries, widows reporting they are engaging in either cash or non-cash generating activities at the time of the census are treated as being economically active. This definition is employed because any activity that materially contributes to the household economies is assumed to increase the status and power of widows within their household of residence. While the majority of elderly widows in this analysis report no economic activity, nearly half of each group (42 percent of Filipinos, 46 percent of Fijians) do offer material contributions to their households.

Disability status also determines the status and power of widowed females within households. While disabled individuals can and do contribute to household economies in a number of ways, these contributions are often limited, and could be offset by the potential costs of medical care and the increased strains on limited household resources. In general, it is assumed that disabled elderly will require higher levels of family support than nondisabled elderly. The reported rates of disability among elderly widows are consistent with rates seen in other nations with Palawan at 11 percent disabled and Fiji at 14 percent disabled. As would be expected, there is a close relationship between disability and economic inactivity, with 73 percent of the disabled Palawan widows and 86 percent of disabled Fijian widows reporting no economic activity.

MULTIVARIATE ANALYSIS MODEL

To measure the effects of age, education, level of economic activity and disability status on the residential structure of elderly female widows, the analysis will employ a multinomial logistic model. Multinomial logistic regression allows for the simultaneous estimation of the relative risks of living in one of the four residential types while controlling for specified demographic and socioeconomic variables. Using the category of widows who live alone as the reference group, the model will estimate the probabilities that elderly female widows are more likely to live in an extended household where they are either the household heads, living with their children or living with others. In line with common practice, the results of the multivariate analysis are presented here as relative risks rather than as regression coefficients; consequently the interpretation of specific variables will be in terms of the increasing or decreasing risks for widows to live in a specific type of extended household relative to their risk of living alone.

RESULTS

General Pooled Model for Residential Choice

Table 2 presents results for the pooled sample of 7,467 widows from Palawan (6,300 widows) and from Vanua Levu (1,167 widows). Age effects are generally moderate to weak for the risk of living with children or living with others as compared to living alone but these risks[1] tend to increase slightly with age as would be expected. While widows aged 65 to 74, for example, have an 8 percent greater risk[2] of living alone compared to widows aged 55 to 64, those aged 75 and older have an 8 percent increased risk of living with children compared to living alone. A similar pattern emerges for the risk of widows to live in the households of others, with widows aged 65 to 74 facing 20 percent greater risk of living alone than the younger widows and those aged 75 and older have a 4 percent greater risk of living with others than living alone. A much stronger negative relationship is seen for the risk of being a household head compared to living alone, with widows aged 64 to 75 facing a 50 percent increased risk of living alone compared to widows aged 55 to 64, and a 63 percent increased risk of living alone if they are aged 75 and older. This suggests that if the elderly widow is unable to associate herself with the home of a child or another individual as she ages, she faces a much greater risk of living alone as opposed to maintaining headship of a complex household.

The effects of completed education on residential choice reflects the pattern of risk associated with a reciprocity model, with poorly educated widows facing increased risks of living alone compared to widows with at least some secondary school education. Compared to widows with a secondary education or more, widows with no formal education face a 61 percent greater risk of living alone than of being the head of a household, a 17 percent increased risk of living alone relative to living with children and an 8 percent increased risk of living alone relative to living with others. The risk of living alone among widows with a grade school education compared to widows with a secondary education is less than that seen for those widows with no education but these women still face a greater risk of living alone than in any of the other residential forms compared to the better educated women.

For widows reporting no economic activity the opposite pattern emerges, with these women having a substantially decreased risk of living alone as opposed to living in other residential forms. The risk of being a household head is two times that of the risk of living alone among

TABLE 2. Pooled Multinomial Logistic Regression of the Relative Risks of Living in Specific Complex Household Types as Opposed to Living Alone: Widowed Females Aged 55 and Older Residing in Palawan, Philippines, and Vanua Levi, Fiji

Variable	Household Head	Lives With Child	Lives With Other
Age 55 to 64 Years (Reference)	*1.00*	*1.00*	*1.00*
	---	---	---
Age 65 to 74 Years	0.50	0.92	0.80
	(0.05)	*(0.10)*	*(0.09)*
Age 75 and Older	0.37	1.08	1.04
	(0.04)	*(0.14)*	*(0.14)*
No Formal Education	0.39	0.83	0.92
	(0.06)	*(0.14)*	*(0.16)*
Grade School Education	0.89	0.94	0.94
	(0.11)	*(0.13)*	*(0.14)*
Secondary or More (Reference)	1.00	1.00	1.00
	---	---	---
No Economic Activity	2.07	14.62	10.88
	(0.21)	*(1.70)*	*(1.32)*
Has Disability	0.69	0.90	0.59
	(0.12)	*(0.22)*	*(0.18)*
Unemployed and Disabled	0.85	0.79	0.98
	(0.22)	*(0.24)*	*(0.35)*
Palawan Widows	0.62	0.18	0.12
	(0.10)	*(0.03)*	*(0.02)*

Standard Errors in italics below Relative Risk Ratios

economically inactive widows, while these women have a 14 times greater risk of living with children and an 11 times greater risk of living with others compared to the risk of living alone. This kind of finding is very much in line with an altruistic model of care where the elderly without resources are taken into extended households. While nothing is known about the level of support these widows are receiving or the economic strength of the households they live in, the ability of the extended household to provide an immediate pool of caregivers in times of need makes it a more desirable residential choice than living alone. Consequently, the finding that the economically weak have a reduced risk of living alone can be interpreted as a positive outcome for widowed females.

In contrast, the risks associated with disability status and residential choice show that disabled widows consistently face higher risk of living alone compared to widows without disabilities. This effect is strongest when they do not live with their children, with disabled widows having a 31 percent greater risk of living alone compared to being household heads and a 41 percent greater risk of living alone compared to living with others. Having children with homes of their own seems to offer a slight advantage to disabled widows, but even here these women face a 10 percent greater risk of living alone compared to widows without disabilities. Similarly, widowed women who are both economically inactive and disabled face a greater risk of living alone than of residing in any form of complex household.

Finally, Table 3 presents a measure testing the overall difference in the relative risks for Filipino widows in Palawan to reside in complex households as compared to Fijian widows in Vanua Levi. In general, widows in Palawan face a uniformly higher risk of living alone than do widows in Vanua Levi. For example, compared to Fijian widows, Filipino widows face an 82 percent greater risk of living alone than of living with their children controlling for other factors. This much higher risk for Palawan widows to live alone suggests that differences that are specific to the independent cultures and economies play a role in the residential outcomes of elderly widows within these study areas.

TABLE 3. Additive Effects for the Pooled Relative Risks of Living in Specific Complex Household Types as Opposed to Living Alone: Widowed Females Aged 55 and Older Residing in Palawan, Philippines, and Vanua Levi, Fiji

	Palawan, Philippines			Vanua Levi, Fiji		
Variables	Head	Lives With Child	Lives With Others	Head	Lives With Child	Lives With Others
Age 65 to 74 Years	0.45	0.08	0.04	0.33	0.60	0.51
Age 75 and Older	0.30	0.09	0.04	0.84	1.94	1.73
No Formal Education	0.32	0.07	0.04	1.01	1.73	1.53
Grade School Education	0.75	0.08	0.75	1.07	0.96	0.85
No Economic Activity	1.67	1.68	0.67	2.65	4.36	3.50
Has Disability	0.58	0.09	0.02	0.73	0.75	0.76
Unemployed and Disabled	0.75	0.06	0.05	0.52	0.81	0.36

Full Pooled Model for Residential Choice

To test for country-specific differences, a full interactive model was run using the pooled data set that controlled for Filipino versus Fijian origin for each of the independent variables. As the relative risks of residential choice for each country-specific site represent the additive effects of the joint model coefficients, the comparative results are summarized in Table 3.[3] To assist in the interpretation of these results, country site specifics are presented graphically in Figures 1 through 3.

Figure 1 presents the comparative risks of residential choice for Filipino and Fijian widows by age. As can be seen in Figure 1, regardless of household type, elderly female widows in Palawan aged 65 to 74 and 75 and older face a uniformly greater risk of living alone than do widows aged 55 to 64 years of age. In contrast, while older Fijian widows have a higher risk of living alone compared to being household heads, for widows who are 75 and older the risk of living with their children is 2 times higher relative to living alone and the risk of living with others is 1.75 times more likely amongst the oldest old. This suggests that while widows aged 65 to 74 have a uniformly greater risk of living alone across the study sites, the opportunities for the oldest old widows differ dramatically between Palawan and Vanua Levu, with Fijian widows having a greater access to the potential benefits obtained from residing in a complex household.

Figure 2 presents the comparative risks of residential choice for Filipino and Fijian widows by educational attainment. It is seen that widows in Palawan with a grade school education or less face marked increases in the risk of living alone relative to widows with a secondary education. Interestingly, the greatest risk of living alone among Filipino widows with low educational attainment is relative to their risk of living with their children. In stark contrast, education effects are much different for the population of Fijian widows. Here, educational attainment plays essentially no role in the risk of being a household head relative to living alone, and the least educated have the greatest opportunities to live either with their children or with others compared to those with a secondary education or more. This kind of finding is generally consistent with the high normative pressures among Fijians to help others and to maintain kinship networks through coresidence and again suggests Fijian widows may obtain access to complex households more easily than widows from Palawan may.

Figure 3 presents the comparative risks of residential choice for Filipino and Fijian widows by economic activity and disability status.

FIGURE 1. Age Effects on Residential Choice Among Elderly Widows Aged 55 and Older: Palawan, Philippines, and Vanua Levu, Fiji—1995 to 1996

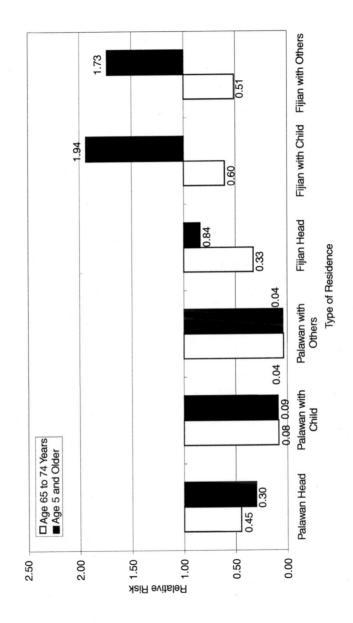

FIGURE 2. Education Effects on Residential Choice Among Elderly Widows Aged 55 and Older: Palawan, Philippines, and Vanua Levu, Fiji–1995 to 1996

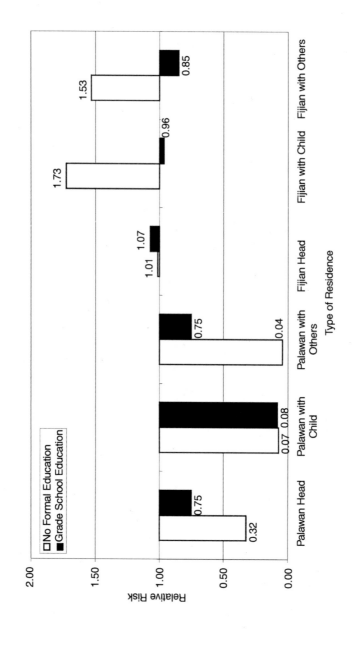

These variables present a consistent pattern and direction regardless of whether the respondent was from Palawan or Vanua Levi, but the magnitudes of the relative risks do vary by country site. Overall, widows who were economically inactive had a lower risk of living alone relative to all other residential types regardless of country. The one exception was for Palawan where widows had a 23 percent greater risk of living alone relative to living with others. In terms of magnitude, Fijian widows who were economically inactive faced a much lower risk of living alone, ranging from a 2.65 higher risk of being a household head to a 4.36 higher risk of living with children as opposed to living alone compared to about a 30 percent decreased risk of living alone among widows in Palawan.

The presence of a disabling condition increases the risk of living alone among both Filipinos and Fijians, but widows in Palawan are at a strikingly increased risk if they are disabled. While being disabled places widows in Palawan at a 25 percent greater risk of living alone relative to being a household head, they have only a 9 percent risk of living in the home of their children and only a 2 percent risk of living with others if they are disabled. In essence, this suggests that disabled widows have little or no chance of entering a complex household they do not control if they have a disabling condition. While Fijian widows also face an increased risk of living alone if they are disabled, the effect is more moderate, with widows facing approximately a 25 percent increased risk of living alone relative to other residential forms. While this is a marked increase in risk, it lacks the magnitude of the impact that disability has upon residential choice among widows in Palawan. When the impacts of being both disabled and economically inactive are examined, increased risks are seen among Fijians for living alone relative to being a household head and living with others but the risk for Fijian widows to live with their children increases slightly. Overall, while economic inactivity does not negatively impact the ability of Filipino and Fijian widows to be part of a complex household, being disabled represents a clear barrier to obtaining the direct forms of caregiving and support that complex households can provide.

DISCUSSION

Elderly female widows represent a risk population of particular concern in the developing world. As many of these women emerged from cultures that discouraged both educational attainment and economic in-

FIGURE 3. Effects of Economic Activity and Disability on Residential Choice Among Elderly Widows Aged 55 and Older: Palawan, Philippines, and Vanua Levu, Fiji—1995 to 1996

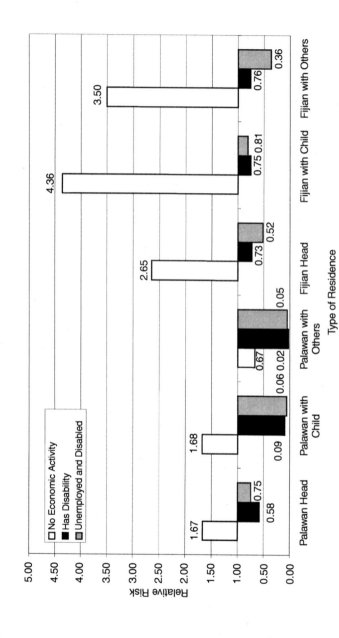

dependence, they often lack the skills and wealth to maintain autonomy and independence in old age. Consequently, elderly widows are typically dependent upon the extended family for support and care in later life. Access to acceptable levels of care are normally expressed in the form of coresidence, either with children or other members of the extended family who are willing to assume the burden of care for the aged household member. Support flows can be bi-directional, with the elderly not only receiving support but also providing services such as childcare, housekeeping or gardening. Eventually, however, age and the increased risks of chronic morbidity can limit the in-kind exchanges the elderly can provide. When this stage of the lifecourse is reached, elderly widows may face increasing levels of unmet need as they can no longer contribute to the household economies upon which they depend.

This paper has examined a specific aspect of the support process by measuring the risks and opportunities for elderly widows to live in one of four household types. In terms of support it was assumed that widows who lived alone were at greatest risk of poverty and unmet need and that widows who lived with children had optimized their available residential choices. To test the broad generalizability of the residential choice model, two independent study sites were selected from sub-regions of the Philippines and Fiji. In broad terms, the patterns of residential choice were driven along expected lines. Younger and better educated widows had the best opportunities to optimize their residential choices, having the lowest risks of living alone.

While somewhat surprising from the perspective of reciprocity, economically inactive elderly widows also had low overall risks of living alone despite their lack of reportable economic contribution to the household economies. While not tested, this may be driven in part by altruistic aspects of Filipino and particularly Fijian culture, but in-kind contributions may also play a role. Healthy but non-job seeking widows often play a major role in household economies through childcare and services such as house cleaning, cooking and light gardening. These services free up the time of younger household members who can then engage in more labor intensive or cash generating activities. While not completely clear from this analysis it is an obvious line of research that needs to be pursued as a result of the present outcomes.

A clear and persistent finding for this study is the impact of disability on the increased risk of living alone. For both the Filipino and Fijian widows, having a disability reduced the chances that they would be able to optimize their residential choices. There are two explanations for this finding. One is that the disabled are typically limited in their ability to provide either economic or in-kind transfers to the household economies and, therefore, in their ability to negotiate access to the potential support services within an extended household. Secondly, the disabled represent cost. Rather than contributing to the household they are a burden both in terms of cash expenses for food, clothing and medicines and in terms of human resources within the household that must be expended for caregiving instead of more profitable activities. It appears the response for both Filipinos and Fijian cultures is to dissociate themselves from the direct residential burden of coresiding with disabled elderly and to allow them to live alone. While qualitative reports in both the Philippines and Fiji suggest that support is often indirectly available to these elderly, it is also clear that the level of support provided is irregular and typically inadequate. From a policy perspective it is clear that the disabled elderly, represent the group at greatest risk of poverty and unmet need and could benefit from targeted programs to assist them.

In general, the situation of elderly female widows is far from dire. The majority continue to live within complex households where they can play a productive role in the household and receive at least minimal support and care. While the family in both Palawan and Vanau Levi appears to be maintaining the brunt of elderly support, as is consistent throughout the developing world, this analysis is also consistent with early work that suggests that as the elderly become older and more frail they also become at risk of abandonment and unmet need for care and support. Longevity increases worldwide have rapidly outpaced the ability of health care systems to deal with chronic impairments related to the aged. As chronic disabilities such as diabetes, hypertension, stroke and dementia become increasingly prevalent in nations such as the Philippines and Fiji, the ability of families to maintain traditional support networks has already become strained. Proactive and guided action is called for if they are to deal with this emerging generation of elderly who can expect not only an increased lifespan but also the potential for increased survivorship with disabling conditions and uncertain support.

NOTES

1. The term *Risk* reflecting merely the positive or negative direction of the relative risk for an event to occur.
2. 8 percent being the inverse of 92 percent.
3. A copy of the full model is available from the author upon request.

REFERENCES

Aghajanian, A. (1985). Living arrangements of widows in Shiraz, Iran. *Journal of Marriage and the Family, 47*, 781-784.

Bowen, E.S. (1964). *Return to laughter.* Garden City, N.Y., Doubleday, 1964.

Cain, M. (1991). Widows, sons, and old-age security in rural Maharashtra: A comment on Vlassoff. *Population Studies, 45*, 519-528.

Cowgill, D.O. (1972). *Aging and modernization.* New York, Appleton-Century-Crofts.

DaVanzo, J. & Chan, A. (1994). Living arrangements of older Malaysians: Who coresides with their adult children? *Demography, 31*, 95-113.

Dwyer, J.W., Lee, G.R., & Jankowski, T.B. (1994). Reciprocity, elder satisfaction, and caregiver stress and burden: The exchange of aid in the family caregiving relationship. *Journal of Marriage and the Family, 56*, 35-43.

Goody J. (1996). Comparing family systems in Europe and Asia: Are there different sets of rules? *Population and Development Review*, 1-20.

Keith, C. (1995). Family caregiving systems: Models, resources, and values. *Journal of Marriage and the Family, 57*, 179-189.

Lillard, L.A. & Willis, R.J. (1997). Motives for intergenerational transfers: Evidence from Malaysia. *Demography, 34*, 115-134.

Martin, L.G. (1989). Living arrangements of the elderly in Fiji, Korea, Malaysia, and the Philippines. *Demography, 26*, 627-643.

_____.(1990). The status of South Asia's growing elderly population. *Journal of Cross Cultural Gerontology*, 593-117.

Mutran, E. & Reitzes, D.C. (1984). Intergenerational support activities and well-being among the elderly: A convergence of exchange and symbolic interaction perspectives. *American Sociological Review, 49*, 117-130.

Nugent, J.B. (1985). The old-age security motive for fertility. *Population and Development Review, 11*, 75-97.

Panapasa, S. (2000). *Sociable security: Family support and elderly well-being in Fiji 1966-1986.* Doctoral dissertation submitted to Brown University.

_____.(2002). Disability among older women and men in Fiji: Concerns for the future. *Journal of Women & Aging, 14* (forthcoming).

Panapasa & McNally, J.W. (1997). "From cradle to grave: Health expectancy and family support among the elderly in the Fiji Islands." Brown University, PSTC Working Paper. WP97-10. August, 1997.

Rasmussen, S.J. (1989). Accounting for belief: Causation, misfortune and evil in Tuareg systems of thought. *Man, 24*, 124-144.

Rensel, J. & Howard, A. (1997). The place of persons with disabilities in Rotuman society. *Pacific Studies, 20*, 19-50.

Williams, L. & Domingo, L. (1993). The social status of elderly women and men within the Filipino family. *Journal of Marriage and the Family, 55*, 415-426.

United Nations. (1999). International year of older persons 1999 proclamation on ageing. A/RES/47/5. 42nd Plenary Meeting. 16 October 1992. United Nations Division for Social Policy and Development.

Vlassoff, C. (1990). The value of sons in an Indian village: How widows see it. *Population Studies, 44*, 5-20.

African Widows:
Anthropological and Historical Perspectives

Maria G. Cattell, PhD

SUMMARY. Variety characterizes widows' experiences around the world and in Africa south of the Sahara. This article explores the socio-economic and cultural contexts of African widowhood, using anthropological studies in a number of African societies, including the author's research among Abaluyia of western Kenya. Some features of African widowhood are characteristic of African women's lives regardless of their marital status: their embeddedness in kinship systems and dependence on those systems for claims to productive resources, their economic self-reliance (which does not mean prosperity), strongly gendered divisions of labor, and the pervasiveness of patriarchal gender relations.

The author is deeply grateful, as always, to her Abaluyia co-researchers, especially John Barasa "JB" Owiti of Samia and Frankline Mahaga of Bunyala and Nairobi, Medical Mission Sisters and Holy Family Hospital at Nangina, Nangina Girls Primary School (now St. Catherine's), and various officials, among others, who made her research possible. The author also thanks the University of Nairobi's Institute of African Studies, where she was a Research Associate (1984-1985), and her late husband Bob Moss. *Mutio muno* to the many people of Samia and Bunyala, and other Luyia people, who have allowed the author to share their lives.

Address correspondence to: Maria G. Cattell, 486 Walnut Hill Road, Millersville, PA 17551-9786.

This research was partially funded by the National Science Foundation (grant BNS8206802), the Wenner-Gren Foundation for Anthropological Research (grant 4506), and Bryn Mawr College (Frederica de Laguna Fund grant).

[Haworth co-indexing entry note]: "African Widows: Anthropological and Historical Perspectives." Cattell, Maria G. Co-published simultaneously in *Journal of Women & Aging* (The Haworth Press, Inc.) Vol. 15, No. 2/3, 2003, pp. 49-66; and: *Widows and Divorcees in Later Life: On Their Own Again* (ed: Carol L. Jenkins) The Haworth Press, Inc., 2003, pp. 49-66. Single or multiple copies of this article are available for a fee from The Haworth Document Delivery Service [1-800-HAWORTH, 9:00 a.m. - 5:00 p.m. (EST). E-mail address: docdelivery@haworthpress.com].

10.1300/J074v15n02_04

49

Other features are specific to widowhood, including remarriage, issues of personal autonomy, and loss of status, access to productive resources and social support. Colonial and postcolonial historical transformations, including Africa's current dire economic situation and the AIDS epidemic, are considered in relation to widows' lives. An interesting question (given the theme of this edited volume) is whether a husband's death puts African widows "on their own again," and whether, given African systems of kinship and marriage, most African women (and indeed men, too) can ever be said to be "on their own." *[Article copies available for a fee from The Haworth Document Delivery Service: 1-800-HAWORTH. E-mail address: <docdelivery@haworthpress.com> Website: <http://www.HaworthPress.com> © 2003 by The Haworth Press, Inc. All rights reserved.]*

KEYWORDS. Africa, Kenya, families, gender, kinship, widows

AFRICAN WIDOWS: A TRUE STORY

Case Study No. 1: Samia of Kenya. Three old widows stay on their husband's land. Manyuru, Aguje and Magoba were co-wives whose husband, a colonial chief, died in 1964. When I met them, in 1984, the three old women were still living on a small portion of his land, each in her own one-room thatch roof house. Aguje's and Magoba's houses, built by their sons, were larger and in better condition than Manyuru's, whose only son was dead. Finally a stepson, son of another of their husband's many wives, built her a new house, small but weather-tight. Once I gave Manyuru a few shillings. She cradled the coins in her hands, smiled and said: "Now I am a woman who is sure, like a woman with a husband." Sure of a meal, she meant! For Manyuru, frail and nearly blind, depended mostly on various stepsons for food and other help. Aguje and Magoba were strong enough to grow their own food which they occasionally shared with Manyuru. Manyuru died in 1992; the other two—with some help from their children—survived until 1995. The three old widows had stayed on their husband's land for over thirty years after his death, secure in their place in their families and secure in their right to cultivate their husband's land.

A SOCIODEMOGRAPHIC OVERVIEW

Similar patterns in the lives of girls and women from birth through old age are found throughout the world (Cattell, 1996a). Females are less highly valued than males, and their work is less highly valued. From infancy through old age females have lesser access than men to resources such as food, education, healthcare, housing, land, livestock, employment and pensions. Women are more likely than men to work in informal sectors of the economy, to earn less, to be poor. Women are more likely than men to be caregivers, to depend on children for old age support, to be childless, to live long enough to become frail. Women have greater longevity than men and are more likely than men to be widowed and to be widows for many years.

Because of spousal age differences, polygyny and greater opportunity for remarriage, relatively few African men, even the oldest, are unmarried. In African countries south of the Sahara, the propositions of men without a wife[1] tend to be in the single digits while the proportions of women who are widows are anywhere from five to nine times greater. In Kenya, for example, only 7% of men age 60 and over are widowed, compared to 50% of women.[2] In 27 African nations with available data, about 42% to 62% of women aged 60 and over are widows (United Nations, 1993).[3]

Of course not all widows are old, but many are. In the absence of much research on African widows, one may (with caution) use information from research on older Africans for characterizing–in very general terms–the situation of widows. The majority of older Africans (women and men) reside in rural areas among kin, many in extended family living arrangements. Like most Africans, they are poor and have little access to healthcare. Many receive support and care from their families. But there are differences. Men who are widowed tend to retain their status and property rights. When a woman is widowed, her social status may drop. Women's claims to resources and family support may be diminished or lost when husbands die. Remarriage may be an issue, though in general older women are much less likely than older men to remarry. However, experiences of widowhood vary widely across the continent, and even in different cultures in the same geographic area–or within one culture. In rural western Kenya, among Gusii (Håkansson, 1994) and Luo (Potash, 1986a), a widow's rights to land are secured through sons, and a woman without sons may lose home and farm on her husband's death. Among Samia people, also in western Kenya, even a widow with no son remains on her husband's land and has the right to a plot to raise food and cash crops for herself and any dependents she has (Case Study No. 1). On the other hand, widows may lose both status and material goods when husbands die, as in Case Study No. 2 (below)–though even here, where most widows struggled for survival, 6% of the widows surveyed said they were being fully supported by someone.

AFRICAN TRANSFORMATIONS, COLONIAL
AND POSTCOLONIAL

During the past several centuries, transformations have occurred–and are continuing–in every aspect of African life. The historical changes in Africa include European colonial domination and exploitation of Africans, the rapid growth of cities and the far-reaching consequences of the introduction of money, wage labor and labor migration, Christianity, and European languages, education, medicine and legal systems–all competing with indigenous ideologies and lifeways. Poverty increased greatly (Iliffe, 1987). Class formation and the development of rural-urban differences in attitudes, activities and lifestyles are also part of the picture. Postcolonial Africa's litany of disasters includes the deepening of individual poverty and national economic downturns brought about by internal corruption, the IMF's structural adjustment programs and the abandonment of Africa by world capitalism (Ferguson, 1999:241-242), increasing political instability and armed conflicts, and the devastations of the AIDS epidemic.

These changes often are referred to by the loosely descriptive term "modernization," usually undefined but cited in many conference papers and publications as the "reason" for the contemporary neglect in Africa of old parents and other vulnerable persons such as widows and the disabled. All too often, these papers and publications lack historical perspective and rely on opinions, assertions, stereotypes and sweeping generalizations as "evidence" for the "disappearance" of the African family and "complete neglect" of elders. This professional discourse is joined to a folk discourse with similar perspectives: in the past elders and others were completely protected by the "traditional" African family, now the family is falling apart (Cattell, 1997b).[4] While there is some truth in these discourses, there is also much exaggeration. African families are not disappearing. They are under stress, they are changing, but they remain the most basic and reliable support system Africans have (e.g., Cattell, 1997c; Ferreira, 1999; Weisner, Bradley and Kilbride, 1997), especially in the absence of viable alternatives such as state welfare and public or private pensions and in the presence of widespread poverty and various unsettling conditions such as war and AIDS.

Although African lifeways, beliefs and values have undergone many dislocations and transformations, African ideologies and customs provide a continuing, though often contested, basis for ordering, interpreting and reinterpreting individual lives.[5] Among African cultural characteristics which are especially important for widows and older people are the salience of seniority and filial obligation in relationships; highly gendered spaces, knowledge, work and opportunities; and the importance of plural marriage, especially polygyny–the marriage of one man to two or more women simultaneously (polyandry occurs in a few African societies).

The following discussion of African widows has a historical aspect, with older ethnographic works taken as a kind of historical baseline.[6] Many ethnographies pay little attention to African widows, but one work (Potash, 1986b) focuses on them, taking a processual approach to try to get at the lived experiences of widows. It is based on research carried out in 11 African societies during the 1960s and 1970s. Potash (1986c) reviewed the rather sparse information on African widows in anthropological research going back to the 1940s (e.g., Cohen, 1969; Evans-Pritchard, 1949; Fortes, 1949; Goody, 1979; Richards, 1951). These ethnographies, written under the functionalist paradigm, focus on institutional arrangements and social rules rather than actual behavior, so their view of widowhood is normative rather than experiential.

Since about the time of publication of Potash's book, poverty has gained a firmer grip on African nations and African individuals, gender violence has increased, armed conflicts have proliferated, the numbers of refugees have increased dramatically, and AIDS has devastated the lives of many Africans. The lives of Africans in general, and of widows in particular, have become much more difficult, with families struggling to meet their obligations to widows and dependent children–and sometimes falling short, sometimes failing altogether. For example, "grabbing" the marital property by the husband's relatives has become common (though not universal) in some areas (Ncube and Stewart, 1995; Owen, 1996).

Case Study No. 2: Shona and Tonga of Zimbabwe. "A woman without a man is not respected." Survey research was conducted in the mid-1980s with older (age 55 and up) Zimbabwean widows, nearly two-thirds having been widows for ten or more years. They lived in subsistence agriculture areas where hard work and poverty characterized the lives of most of them. Of the 270 widows in the study, only 20% received any substantial property inheritance from their husband's estate. Though 62% remained in their homes, some had only minimal goods (a few pots and dishes, a blanket or two, a hoe), their in-laws having "grabbed" the rest. Nearly half the women (48%) were responsible for children, grandchildren and/or other family. Most stated that they were much worse off economically as widows than they had been as wives; getting adequate food was their major problem. Although many had made sacrifices to educate their children, only 48% reported receiving financial assistance from their children. About a fifth of the widows remarried, apparently by their own choice, though many of the remarried widows discovered that the new husband was only after their worldly goods. Many of the women felt abandoned, abused, not respected (Compiled from Folta and Deck, 1987).

SOCIOECONOMIC AND CULTURAL CONTEXTS OF WIDOWHOOD

The experiences of African widows grow out of the socioeconomic, political and cultural contexts of African marriage and women's roles as wives. How marriages are established, where wives live, their access to productive resources and other economic opportunities, who "owns" children, women's rights in their natal kin groups, mourning practices and the degree to which they restrict widows in their ordinary activities, remarriage options, who provides material support and caregiving–all these are among the factors influencing the lives of African widows. Each widow's life is shaped within a particular sociocultural matrix (though even within one culture there is variation and room for maneuvering) and refined by personal factors such as her personality, relationships with her in-laws, whether bridewealth was paid fully, in part or not at all, her mourning behavior and her own economic resources. Thus widowhood is a sociocultural construction elaborated by the widow's in-laws, who decide whether her marriage was valid and what actions to take for or against the widow, and the woman's perceptions of herself as a widow and what she can do, what she must accept.

Access to agricultural land is crucial to the survival of the majority of Africans, who live in rural areas and are peasant farmers growing both subsistence and cash crops. Few African women own land; they depend on usufruct (use) rights to agricultural land through kinship connections, most commonly husbands,[7] who allocate fields for their wives' use and usually are responsible for building houses. Families are the basic producing units in this "familial mode of production" (Caldwell, 1982), a more reliable means (along with informal sector activities) to survival than dependence on the market economy (Gordon, 1995). Growing competition for ever-scarcer economic resources promotes the family mode of production, since it allows a greater range of claims to resources among various kin;[8] the competition also encourages efforts to restrict even further women's economic opportunities (Gordon,

1995). Following a husband's death, some widows retain their cultivation and residential rights, as among Abaluyia of Kenya (Case Study No. 1; Cattell, 1997a). In other Kenyan groups, including Gusii (Håkansson, 1994), Luo (Potash, 1986a) and Nandi (Oboler, 1986), widows' rights to land come through sons. These widows often manage their sons' estates until they decide to retire, after which sons provide for mothers. Potash (1986a) found in her 1970s research that most Luo widows continued to reside in their marital homes and were supported by sons. However, especially in the current economic climate, some widows (among Luo and in many other ethnic groups) may be dispossessed, driven off their husband's land and left to fend for themselves–actions justified by strongly held beliefs that a man's heirs are his kin, not his wife, and maybe not even his children (Case Studies 2 and 3; Ncube and Stewart, 1995; Owen, 1996).

Case Study No. 3: On the Zambian Copperbelt. Violence against wives and widows. Since the 1930s, copper provided much of Zambia's wealth. Mineworkers and their families prospered. But the severe economic downturn of the past two decades has brought deep poverty to the Copperbelt. It has intensified the misogyny of mineworkers and the antagonisms common in conjugal and quasi-conjugal relationships in which women (most have very little earning power) exchange sexual and domestic services for economic support from men. Violence and sexual infidelity (of women and men) often characterize these relationships; many are temporary. If a man retires to his home village where his wife is an outsider, she is likely to be met with hostility from his kin. She may be accused of "witchcraft" (injuring or killing others by beatings and poison) or be the victim of it–but witchcraft is endemic, practiced not just against widows, but also against neighbors and kin, especially anyone who appears to be more prosperous. Husbands' kin routinely take all household property from widows, for they believe that the heirs of a deceased man are his matrilineal kin, not his spouse or children. This violence, while particularly harsh against widows, is rooted in both matrilineal ideologies and the current abysmal political economy of Zambia (Compiled from Ferguson, 1999).

In African societies kinship shapes identities and life choices in many ways. In most African societies, descent groups (some numbering in the thousands) are patrilineal, reckoning descent, inheritance and positional succession through males. Women usually leave their natal homes to reside in the husband's home and are generally regarded as outsiders to the family. Often, having no right to return to their natal group, widows in patrilineal groups have little choice but to remain with the husband's family (unless the family rejects her) in order to have access to productive resources and be with her children (who belong to the father's family) (e.g., Potash, 1986c). Matrilineal societies, reckoning descent and inheritance through females, offer important advantages to women, who often have strong rights in their natal group. Some communities develop around groups of related women for whom widowhood does not change their rights of residence; in other matrilineal groups, women retain the right to return to their natal groups when they are widowed, or even before, if they decide to "retire" from marriage (e.g., Stucki, 1992). Women among matrilineal Ndembu of Zambia ordinarily return to their natal groups when their children are grown, even if their husbands are alive, and mature sons reside with their mothers no matter where she chooses to live (Turner, 1957). Some societies are bilineal (cognatic, duolineal)–both maternal and paternal kinship are important (Etienne, 1986).

Throughout sub-Saharan Africa women are jural minors, under the control of males (fathers, brothers and husbands) and unable to act legally on their own account. Property, even when modern legal systems allow for inheritance by females, generally goes to males, the primary exception being Muslim groups, where a man's widows and daughters do inherit property, though a smaller portion than sons. African women are the primary producers of both cash and subsistence crops (though they do not always control the products of their labor) and are expected to contribute substantially to household economies. Reproduction–the bearing and raising of children–and household maintenance (domestic) activities are almost exclusively women's work. The demands of these activities, along with educational disadvantages and persisting patterns of patriarchal oppression (indigenous and colonial), have severely limited African women's roles in the formal economy, leading to heavy participation in the informal economy, especially as micro-entrepreneurs. In addition, serious health consequences result from pronatalism and lack of reproductive freedom which lead to multiple pregnancies among women who are overworked and very poor.[9]

Nevertheless, as Potash (1986c) points out, African widows generally have alternatives. They have options for their futures, though they also have constraints on what they can do, including the "ordinary" constraints of African women (previous paragraph) and the special constraints placed on widows. The choices and constraints vary across the continent and even within a single ethnic community. "Customs" or "tradition" are invoked as behavioral norms, yet often are ignored, broken, revised and reinvented in the struggle for survival and accumulation. For example, leviratic marriage (marrying a husband's kinsman to get more children for the deceased husband) is the cultural ideal among Nandi of Kenya, but very few Nandi widows accept a levir. With secure rights in their husband's estates (which will be inherited by their sons), Nandi widows prefer their independence (Oboler, 1986). By contrast, the levirate is technically prohibited among Baule of Cote d'Ivoire, but it is sometimes practiced (Etienne, 1986). In Somalia, religious (Koranic) and cultural rules prescribe the inheritance of land and livestock by daughters and wives, but females rarely inherit. By breaking the rules Somali men retain maximal control of resources. That makes it difficult for Somali women to acquire productive resources, though a few do. The result is that most older widows, with low status and little or no property, depend entirely on support from their children (younger widows usually remarry) (Glascock, 1985, N.d.; cf. Andretta, 1983, on Murle widows in Sudan).

Case Study No. 4: Irigwe and Rukuba of Nigeria. Widows with many choices. Among the polyandrous Rukuba and Irigwe, wives decide with which husband to reside and for how long, and as widows have similar freedom of residential choice and secure rights to land use in each of their marital homes–a degree of matrimonial and postmatrimonial freedom and independence rare in African societies. Widows (like wives) make their choices according to their perceptions of the best deal for themselves, and they can change their minds freely. For Rukuba women, for example, widowhood does not seem to be a critical status except in agricultural production, where husband and wife together can grow more millet than either alone. In the home where she chooses to live, the widow is the head of her household. She manages the marriages of her sons and daughters and (with her co-wives, if she has any in that home) her dead husband's estate. She may take a lover with whom there are no mutual obligations. If all that does not suit her, she may return to the home of another husband or marry yet another man. Older widows are likely to make their choice of residence based on the sons with whom they prefer to live and on whom they will depend for support and care when they can no longer work. (Compiled from Muller, 1986, on Rukuba, and Sangree, 1992, on Irigwe)

WIDOWS' SPECIAL PROBLEMS AND CONCERNS

African widows' many problems and concerns include status loss, economic security, their children's welfare, male domination, remarriage, gender violence, including beatings and rape, witchcraft, and AIDS and other STDs. The AIDS epidemic has greatly increased the number of widows, and these "AIDS widows" (often HIV-infected themselves) are likely to be stigmatized and shunned in their communities and left on their own to cope with supporting themselves and their children.[10] When the widows die, their orphaned children may have only a widowed grandmother to care for them (some call AIDS the "grandmother's disease") or may have to look after themselves. Unknown numbers of widows are refugees, a circumstance which puts them (and all girls and women who are refugees) at tremendous risk of abuse, rape and discrimination in food distributions, training programs and resettlement (Owen, 1996). In some communities, the restrictions and humiliations of mourning practices make life difficult and even force women to leave employment (Ncube and Stewart, 1995; Owen, 1996). Ritual cleansing through sexual intercourse, often amounting to rape, can leave a widow psychologically traumatized, pregnant and/or with an STD. Widows may also be accused of witchcraft and having caused their husbands' death, and may be beaten as a result.[11]

Economic security is a major concern of most African widows. It is closely allied to their responsibilities as mothers and grandmothers. In a situation of widespread poverty, many women (wives and widows) are poor and constantly struggling to make ends meet. African nations are also poor, so public welfare and pensions are rarely available. Even widows eligible for a pension are likely to receive only a minimal lump sum payment–and only after hassling with bureaucrats and waiting for a long time, even for years. Many widows run into difficulties when they no longer have monetary or labor support (however minimal) from husbands, or if their property has been "grabbed" by the husband's relatives or they have been chased from his land (Case Studies No. 2 and 3; Ncube and Stewart, 1995; Owen, 1996). Widows in such circumstances, especially if they have dependent children, are likely to accept remarriage in one of the various conjugal or quasi-conjugal options for widows, including the levirate, widow inheritance, woman-woman marriage and "ordinary" marriage as defined in each culture (see Note 1).

Case Study No. 5: Luo of Kenya. Widows as "wives of the grave." Luo women whose husbands die are *chi liel*, "wives of the grave." They are still married: "It is just bad luck the husband died." Most Luo widows accept a leviratic "husband." The widow chooses the levir from her husband's kin. She stays on her husband's land, in her own house, managing the farm and livestock if her sons are too young to do it. The levir does not reside with nor support her or her children. His only obligation is to father children on behalf of the dead husband. If the widow is past childbearing, the levir's role is merely symbolic. In either case, the wife of the grave is free to manage her own affairs or to turn the farm management over to an adult son, counting on her close ties with him to insure her support. (Sonless women have problems, but relatively few women lack a son.) A Luo wife of the grave is likely to have more economic power and personal autonomy than she had as wife of a living husband (compiled from Potash, 1986a).

Potash (1986c:28) notes that one of the most consistent findings in her volume is "the degree to which [African] widows are economically self-reliant." This is also true of African wives. Self-reliance does not mean prosperity. It means women contribute substantially to their households and may even have primary responsibility for feeding, clothing and meeting healthcare and educational expenses of children and, in many cases, grandchildren. This happens for various reasons, including cultural expectations, insufficient support from husbands, and absence of husbands for employment, sometimes for long periods, as in southern Africa where men work in the gold and diamond mines far from their homes. Migrant labor patterns make many African women de facto household heads. In Ghana and Nigeria, women traders have considerable economic and personal autonomy and commonly are the main support of their households; for them, widowhood is not an economic problem (e.g., Clark, 1994; Ufomata, 1998). For many African women, widowhood as a "permanent status of some independence" (Korieh, 1996:57) is preferable to remarriage. As one Ghanaian woman in her sixties put it: "I have had so much of this bossing by men. . . . I have my house, my garden; I grow my vegetables; I sell in the market. Everything I make is mine. Why should I have a man take it from me, spend my money on drink and other women, or tell me now what to do? I am the boss now" (quoted in Owen, 1996:108).

Among Abaluyia of Kenya, older women, married or not, get more respect and have more decision-making power and control of others' labor than younger women (Cattell, 2002b). They may gain further status as community health workers, certified midwives and religious leaders. As widows, many women consider themselves to be the "owners" (managers) of the home–as few married women do–and assume greater leadership roles in their families. Like West African market women and Luo widows, many Abaluyia widows, especially older women, find they have greater freedom and power without a husband (Cattell, 1996b). While the cultural rule among Abaluyia is that a widow should be "inherited" as a wife by the dead husband's kinsman,[12] in practice it did not always happen in the past and, especially with older widows, was primarily for ritual purposes to clear the pollution of death (Whyte, 1990). Today, widow inheritance appears to be declining among Abaluyia as more widows are refusing it. Among the Samia and Banyala subgroups of Abaluyia, many widows rationalize their refusal in terms of their religious beliefs as born-again Christians (Cattell, 1992). Women are also explicit that they do not want another husband: "when you get a man you have to take care of him" or "a man would just eat my food" (be a consumer, not a contributor).

Case Study No. 6: Samia of Kenya. "Men would just eat me." Florence was in her early forties when her husband died, in 1994, leaving her with eight children to raise on her own. After the burial, she stayed on her husband's land, in the modern house they had built. Florence is a hardworking farmer who grows much of her own food and also owns a cow her brothers gave her. In addition, she has a job at a nearby hospital. In June 1995 (only six months after her husband's death) I asked her: "Are you going to be inherited?" "No! I chase the brothers-in-law away," she replied, vehemently. "Men would just eat me. They know I have a job and that is their aim. They would come and eat and contribute nothing." Florence is a strong woman, educated and articulate. She is also supported by her mother-in-law, an equally strong woman. Both women are saved Christians and get support from other saved people. Four years later Florence was still refusing the brothers-in-law (Cattell, 1992, 2002c).

In another Luyia subgroup, the Maragoli, widow inheritance is also declining as some widows refuse it for various reasons involving self-interest, concerns to safeguard property and children, not wanting an abusive or alcoholic husband, religious reasons and wanting to make one's own decisions (Gwako, 1998). Maragoli widows who accepted a husband had similar concerns about their self-interest and their children, but saw their best interests being met by acceptance; family pressures also played a part. Some inherited widows later terminated the relationship because the husband was alcoholic, abusive, misused the household's goods, infected the widow with an STD, and for other reasons. Clearly, there is a growing resistance by African women to patriarchal domination (cf. Abwunza, 1997; Cattell, 1992).

There are alternatives to husbands. Co-wives may help each other (Case Study No. 1). A woman's natal group, especially in matrilineal societies, may be a source of support through various mechanisms, including her return, as a widow or as a "retired" wife, to her home village and matrilineal kin (e.g., Stucki, 1992). But even in some patrilineal societies such as Abaluyia, the natal group may provide help, like Florence's brothers who gave her a cow (Case Study No. 6). In Muslim societies such as the Hausa of Nigeria and Swahili of the East African coast, divorce and remarriage are common throughout life. Women have a great deal of choice in marriage decisions, including the decision not to be married–especially if it interferes with their business (married women usually are secluded, making it difficult to conduct business; widows are not secluded). Their decisions are also influenced by bilateral kinship systems with strong ties among maternal kin and inheritance of property by females as set forth by Sharia (Islamic law) (Coles, 1990; Landberg, 1986; Schildkrout, 1986). African women, married or not, have a high dependence on sons, and often daughters as well, for support and personal care. Mother-son and mother-daughter bonds are often of greater emotional salience than marital bonds. They are also of greater practical value in regard to care in old age, since husbands do not provide personal care, but daughters and daughters-in-law do.

AFRICAN WIDOWS: ON THEIR OWN AGAIN?

This discussion has included dire extremes of widowhood and instances where women are better off as widows than they were as wives. The extent of African widows' experiences–how many have which kind of experience–is unknown, except we know that the lives of most Africans, male and female, are difficult, or "miserable" as Kenyan women's activist Wangari Maathai put it (quoted in Gordon, 1995, 883).[13] But even allowing that men, too, participate in misery, they have far and away the better of it when it comes to patriarchal gender relations and economic opportunity.

There is no "typical" African widow. Each woman's experiences are uniquely her own, and even within a given sociocultural framework, widows have very different experiences. Culture and kinship–highly subjective and flexible–are invoked and reinterpreted, negotiated and reimagined as individuals struggle to survive and to maximize their opportunities. Few of these struggles achieve the flamboyance and notoriety of Wambui Otieno's attempt to escape from culture and kinship when her husband died (Gordon, 1995; Stamp, 1991). Wambui was able to make the attempt, though in the end her escape was only partial; but most African widows, lacking Wambui's skills, wealth and power, remain embedded in the kin groups and cultural modalities that structure their lives from birth. And the "miserable men" are right there with them.

So, are African widows "on their own again"? Not really. Few Africans are ever on their own. Many widows may be on their own financially–but they may have been on their own as wives: the main support of their families, the managers of children, farms and kitchens. They know how to get along, within the constraints imposed on them by poverty and patriarchy. Even the widow rejected by her husband's family is likely to have at least a few (and perhaps many) of her own kin to turn to; they may or may not be able to help her materially, but the connections are there. Being on your own is on the outer limits of possibility for most Africans–including widows.

NOTES

1. I say "men without a wife" because polygyny (widespread in some parts of Africa) means that a man can lose one wife (or more) and yet remain married. Is such a man a widower? Is he perhaps a widower for the duration of a short mourning period during which he is supposed to–but doesn't necessarily–abstain from sex with his other wife or wives? Since, for many women, widow becomes a permanent status, their status might seem clearcut. Yet is "widow" an indigenous African category? Some African "widows" who were "remarried" (in leviratic or "widow inheritance" marriages) do not identify themselves as wives, some do (this happened in my research in Kenya, see Cattell, 1989). Many researchers in Zambia have commented on the ambiguities of "marriage" on the Copperbelt (see Ferguson, 1999). In some African societies, women "retire" from marriage in old age (e.g., Stucki, 1992), or a childless or sonless widow may marry another woman ("woman-woman marriage") or even marry her daughter to the centerpost of her house in order to get children (e.g., Oboler, 1985). Vellenga (1986) reports a list (used in a speech in 1960) of 24 kinds of heterosexual relationships among Akan of Ghana. Surely some of the "problems" in identifying widows are the result of trying to shoehorn African conjugality into Euroamerican social science categories. These ambiguities also raise questions about sociological and anthropological gender categories (Amadiume, 1987; Oboler, 1980).

2. For more demographic details, see Cattell (1997a).

3. Such data must be taken with some salt, since many African elders, especially women, are illiterate and do not know their chronological age, not to mention the difficulties of doing censuses and surveys in nations whose populations are largely rural and whose infrastructure makes travel and communication difficult.

4. As African cultures have been challenged by, and increasingly are challenging, European ideologies and systems, the resulting tensions have frequently been categorized in dichotomies such as "traditional/modern" or "rural/urban." These dichotomies provide too limited a picture, for the spectrum of African life and thought includes more variation and complexity than can be encompassed by such dualisms (cf. Ferguson, 1999).

5. This is not special to Africans; people everywhere manipulate their cultural beliefs, norms and values. Culture is not a straitjacket; it is flexible and negotiable, a rich resource for living.

6. This is a very rough and general "baseline." But the chapters in Potash (1986a) and her excellent discussion (Potash, 1986b) do represent a more prosperous, pre-AIDS era in Africa when the customs calling for protection and care of widows and other vulnerable persons probably operated with a much higher degree of success than they do–or can–now (cf. Iliffe, 1987).

7. In matrilineal societies women may have claims to land and houses through their matriclans, and husbands may have claims to land through their wives–among other possibilities.

8. Gordon (1995, 887) notes that a lineage is like a "court of claims" and determines access to productive resources and other entitlements, and thus is the basis of both production and distribution.

9. On the lives of African women, see, for example, Beneria and Sen (1986), Boserup (1970), Bryceson (1995), Cattell (2002a), Robertson and Berger (1986), Stichter and Parpart (1988), Turshen (1991).

10. One can scarcely overstate the impacts of AIDS in sub-Saharan Africa. In the hardest hit countries, as much as 25% of the adult population is HIV positive. AIDS has reversed declines in infant mortality rates and lowered life expectancies at birth by as much as 20 years in some countries (Ferreira, 2000). African women are especially vulnerable because of their poor health status; women have higher rates of infection and shorter latency periods than men (Owen, 1996).

11. Beating females is commonly accepted in African cultures, for example, husbands may, indeed should beat their wives to teach them proper behavior. Responding to the question, "What do you fear most?" most eighth grade schoolgirls in western Kenya said "beatings" (author's research).

12. Widow inheritance (or "husband succession") is based on the principle that, through the reciprocal rights and obligations established by payment of bridewealth to a woman's kin, the woman becomes the wife of the lineage; if her first husband dies, he should be succeeded as husband by one of his male kin (unless her family returns the bridewealth–which rarely happens).

13. Maathai said: "[Q]uite often we forget that these miserable women are married to miserable men. They are oppressed together."

REFERENCES

Abwunza, Judith M. (1997) *Women's voices, women's power: Dialogues of resistance from East Africa.* Peterborough, Canada: Broadview Press.

Amadiume, Ifi (1987) *Male daughters, female husbands: Gender and sex in an African society.* London: Zed Books.

Andretta, Elizabeth H. (1982) Aging, power and status in an East African pastoral society. In Jay Sokolovsky (Ed.), "Aging and the aged in the Third World, Part II: Regional and ethnographic perspectives," *Studies in Third World Societies,* 23, 83-109.

Beneria, Lourdes and Sen, Gita (1986) Accumulation, reproduction, and women's role in economic development: Boserup revisited. In Eleanor Leacock and Helen I. Safa (Eds.), *Women's work: Development and the division of labor by gender* (pp. 141-157). South Hadley: Bergin & Garvey.

Boserup, Ester (1970) *Woman's role in economic development*. New York: St. Martin's Press.

Bryceson, Deborah Fahey (Ed.) (1995) *Women wielding the hoe: Lessons from rural Africa for feminist theory and development practice*. Oxford: Berg.

Caldwell, John C. (1982) *Theory of fertility decline*. New York: Academic.

Cattell, Maria G. (1989) *Old age in rural Kenya: Gender, the life course and social change*. (Doctoral dissertation, Bryn Mawr College, 1989). University Microfilms No. 9000504.

Cattell, Maria G. (1992) Praise the Lord and say no to men: Older Samia women empowering themselves. *Journal of Cross-Cultural Gerontology*, 7, 307-330

Cattell, Maria G. (1996a) Gender, aging and health: A comparative approach. In Carolyn Sargent and Caroline B. Brettell (Eds.), *Gender and health: An international perspective* (pp. 87-122). Upper Saddle River: Prentice Hall.

Cattell, Maria G. (1996b) Does marital status matter? Support, personal autonomy and economic power among Abaluyia widows in Kenya. *Southern African Journal of Gerontology*, 5(2), 20-26.

Cattell, Maria G. (1997a) African widows, culture and social change: Case studies from Kenya. In Jay Sokolovsky (Ed.), *The cultural context of aging: Worldwide perspectives*, 2nd ed. (pp. 71-98). Westport: Bergin & Garvey.

Cattell, Maria G. (1997b) The discourse of neglect: Family support for the elderly in Samia. In Thomas S. Weisner, Candice Bradley and Philip L. Kilbride (Eds.), *African families and the crisis of social change* (pp. 157-183). Westport: Bergin & Garvey.

Cattell, Maria G. (1997c) Ubuntu, African elderly and the African family crisis. *Southern African Journal of Gerontology*, 6(2), 37-39.

Cattell, Maria G. (2002a) Holding up the sky: Gender, age and work among Abaluyia of Kenya. In Sinfree Makoni and Koenraad Stroeken (Eds.), *Ageing in Africa: Sociolinguistic and anthropological approaches* (pp. 157-177). Aldershot, England: Ashgate.

Cattell, Maria G. (2002b) Gender, age and power: Hierarchy and liminality among Abaluyia women of Kenya. In Mario I. Aguilar (Ed.), *Rethinking age in Africa: Colonial, postcolonial and contemporary interpretations*. Trenton: Africa World Press.

Cattell, Maria G. (2002c) "Men would just eat me": A widow's tale. Short story read at annual meeting of the American Anthropological Association, New Orleans.

Clark, Gracia (1994) *Onions are my husband: Survival and accumulation by West African market women*. Chicago: University of Chicago Press.

Cohen, Abner (1969) *Custom and politics in urban Africa*. Berkeley: University of California Press.

Coles, Catherine (1990) The older woman in Hausa society: Power and authority in urban Nigeria. In Jay Sokolovsky (Ed.), *The cultural context of aging: Worldwide perspectives* (pp. 56-81). New York: Bergin & Garvey.

Etienne, Mona (1986) Contradictions, constraints, and choices: Widow remarriage among the Baule of Ivory Coast. In Betty Potash (Ed.), *Widows in African societies: Choices and constraints* (pp. 241-282). Stanford: Stanford University Press.

Evans-Pritchard, E. E. (1951) *Kinship and marriage among the Nuer.* Oxford: Clarendon Press.

Ferguson, James (1999) *Expectations of modernity: Myths and meanings of urban life on the Zambian Copperbelt.* Berkeley: University of California Press.

Ferreira, Monica (1999) Building and advancing African gerontology. *Southern African Journal of Gerontology,* 8(1), 1-3.

Ferreira, Monica (2000) AIDS–the mad-dog curse of Africa. *Southern African Journal of Gerontology,* 9(1), 1-3.

Folta, Jeannette R. and Deck, Edith S. (1987) Elderly black widows in rural Zimbabwe. *Journal of Cross-Cultural Gerontology,* 2, 321-344.

Fortes, Meyer (1949) *The web of kinship among the Tallensi.* London: Oxford University Press.

Glascock, Anthony P. (1985) Old rules are made to be broken: Resource transfer among agro-pastoralists in Somalia. In John H. Morgan (Ed.), *Aging in developing societies: A reader in Third World gerontology,* Vol. 2 (pp. 61-76).

Glascock, Anthony P. (N.d.) Broken rules and broken promises: Status and role of widows in southern Somalia. Manuscript in author's possession.

Goody, Esther (1973) *Contexts of kinship.* Cambridge: Cambridge University Press.

Gordon, April (1995) Gender, ethnicity, and class in Kenya: "Burying Otieno" revisited. *Signs: Journal of Women in Culture and Society,* 20, 883-912.

Gwako, Edwins Laban Moogi (1998) Widow inheritance among the Maragoli of western Kenya. *Journal of Anthropological Research,* 54, 173-198.

Håkansson, N. Thomas (1994) The detachability of women: Gender and kinship in processes of socioeconomic change among the Gusii of Kenya. *American Ethnologist,* 21, 516-538.

Iliffe, John (1987) *The African poor: A history.* New York: Cambridge University Press.

Korieh, Chima Jacob (1996) *Widowhood among the Igbo of Eastern Nigeria.* M.Phil. thesis, University of Bergen, Norway.

Landberg, Pamela (1986) Widows and divorced women in Swahili society. In Betty Potash (Ed.), *Widows in African societies: Choices and constraints* (pp. 107-130). Stanford: Stanford University Press.

Muller, Jean-Claude (1986) Where to live? Widows' choices among the Rukuba. In Betty Potash (Ed.), *Widows in African societies: Choices and constraints* (pp. 175-192). Stanford: Stanford University Press.

Ncube, Welshman and Stewart, Julie (Eds.) (1995) *Widowhood, inheritance laws, customs & practices in southern Africa.* Harare, Zimbabwe: Women and the Law in Southern Africa Research Project.

Oboler, Regina Smith (1980) Is the female husband a man?: Woman/woman marriage among the Nandi of Kenya. *Ethnology,* 19:69-88.

Oboler, Regina Smith (1985) *Women, power, and economic change: The Nandi of Kenya.* Stanford: Stanford University Press.

Oboler, Regina (1986) Nandi widows. In Betty Potash (Ed.), *Widows in African societies: Choices and constraints* (pp. 66-83). Stanford: Stanford University Press.

Owen, Margaret (1996) *A world of widows.* London: Zed Books.

Potash, Betty (1986a) Wives of the grave: Widows in a rural Luo community. In Betty Potash (Ed.), *Widows in African societies: Choices and constraints* (pp. 44-65). Stanford: Stanford University Press.

Potash, Betty (Ed.) (1986b) *Widows in African societies: Choices and constraints.* Stanford: Stanford University Press.

Potash, Betty (1986c) Widows in Africa: An introduction. In Betty Potash (Ed.), *Widows in African societies: Choices and constraints* (pp. 1-43). Stanford: Stanford University Press.

Richards, Audrey (1951) The Bemba of north-eastern Rhodesia. In Elizabeth Colson and Max Gluckman (Eds.), *Seven tribes of British central Africa.* Oxford: Oxford University Press.

Robertson, Claire and Berger, Iris (Eds.) (1986) *Women and class in Africa.* New York: Africana Publishing Co.

Sangree, Walter H. (1992) Grandparenthood and modernization: The changing status of male and female elders in Tiriki, Kenya, and Irigwe, Nigeria. *Journal of Cross-Cultural Gerontology,* 7, 331-361.

Schildkrout, Enid (1986) Widows in Hausa society: Ritual phase or social state? In Betty Potash (Ed.), *Widows in African societies: Choices and constraints* (pp. 131-152). Stanford: Stanford University Press.

Stamp, Patricia (1991) Burying Otieno: The politics of gender and ethnicity in Kenya. *Signs: Journal of Women in Culture and Society,* 16, 808-845.

Stichter, Sharon B. and Parpart, Jane L. (Eds.) (1988) *Patriarchy and class: African women in the home and the workforce.* Boulder: Westview.

Stucki, Barbara R. (1992) The long voyage home: Return migration among aging cocoa farmers of Ghana. *Journal of Cross-Cultural Gerontology,* 7, 363-378.

Turner, Victor (1957) *Schism and continuity in an African society.* Manchester: Manchester University Press.

Turshen, Meredeth (Ed.) (1991) *Women and health in Africa.* Trenton: Africa World Press.

Ufomata, Titilayo (1998) *Voices from the marketplace.* Ibadan, Nigeria: Kraftgriots.

United Nations (1993) *Demographic yearbook: Population ageing and the situation of elderly people.* New York: United Nations.

Vellenga, Dorothy Dee (1986) The widow among the matrilineal Akan of southern Ghana. In Betty Potash (Ed.), *Widows in African societies: Choices and constraints* (pp. 220-240). Stanford: Stanford University Press.

Weisner, Thomas S., Bradley, Candice, and Kilbride, Philip L. (Eds.) (1997) *African families and the crisis of social change.* Westport: Bergin & Garvey.

Whyte, Susan Reynolds (1990) The widow's dream: Sex and death in western Kenya. In Michael Jackson and Ivan Karps (Eds.), *Personhood and agency: The experience of self and other in African cultures* (pp. 95-114). Uppsala Studies in Cultural Anthropology 14. Stockholm: Almqvist & Wiksell and Washington DC: Smithsonian Institution.

The Impact of Minority Group Status on the Projected Retirement Income of Divorced Women in the Baby Boom Cohort

Barbara A. Butrica, PhD
Howard M. Iams, PhD

SUMMARY. Using projections from the Social Security Administration's Modeling Income in the Near Term (MINT1), we examine the characteristics and retirement income of white non-Hispanic, black non-Hispanic, and Hispanic divorced women in the baby boom cohort. Although we find significant differences in retirement income for divorced women of different racial and ethnic groups, the characteristics associated with higher or lower retirement income are very similar. That

The authors are grateful to Karen Smith and David Wittenburg for helpful discussions and comments.

Address correspondence to: Barbara Butrica, The Urban Institute, 2100 M Street, NW, Washington, DC 20037.

The views in this paper are the authors' only and should not be construed as representing the opinion or policy of The Urban Institute, its Board, or its Sponsors, or the Social Security Administration. The authors had equal responsibility for this work.

This paper was first presented at the Population Association of America Meeting held in Washington, DC, in March 2001.

[Haworth co-indexing entry note]: "The Impact of Minority Group Status on the Projected Retirement Income of Divorced Women in the Baby Boom Cohort." Butrica, Barbara A., and Howard M. Iams. Co-published simultaneously in *Journal of Women & Aging* (The Haworth Press, Inc.) Vol. 15, No. 2/3, 2003, pp. 67-88; and: *Widows and Divorcees in Later Life: On Their Own Again* (ed: Carol L. Jenkins) The Haworth Press, Inc., 2003, pp. 67-88. Single or multiple copies of this article are available for a fee from The Haworth Document Delivery Service [1-800-HAWORTH, 9:00 a.m. - 5:00 p.m. (EST). E-mail address: docdelivery@haworthpress.com].

is, being college educated, owning a home, and having pension and asset income, for example, correspond to increased retirement income for all racial and ethnic groups. However, because black and Hispanic women are less likely than white women to be college educated, to own their home, and to have pension and asset income, their retirement income tends to be lower than that of white women. We conclude the paper by briefly discussing policy options to address the retirement needs of divorced women. *[Article copies available for a fee from The Haworth Document Delivery Service: 1-800-HAWORTH. E-mail address: <docdelivery@haworthpress. com> Website: <http://www.HaworthPress.com>* © *2003 by The Haworth Press, Inc. All rights reserved.]*

KEYWORDS. Women, retirement, aging, race, ethnicity, minority, marital status, divorce, income, economic well-being

INTRODUCTION

In recent years, it has become increasingly common for people to wait until older ages to marry for the first time. Furthermore, many of those who marry will eventually divorce (Ahlburg & De Vita, 1992; Norton & Miller, 1992; DaVanzo & Rahman, 1993; Goldstein, 1999). Although most people who divorce will remarry, the remarriage rate has decreased, and second marriages also often end in divorce (Norton & Miller, 1992).

These trends in marriage, combined with decreasing death rates, suggest that future retirees are more likely to be never married or divorced and less likely to be married or widowed. Unmarried retirees, particularly women, have poverty rates that are much higher than those of married retirees. Among current retirees (65 or older), poverty rates of married women are only 4.4% compared with 23.1% for never married women, 20.3% for divorced women, and 16.5% for widows (Table 8.1 in Grad, 2002).

Our previous work documented the projected economic well-being of future cohorts of divorced women at retirement (Butrica & Iams, 2000). We found large differences in the retirement income and poverty of divorced women that corresponded with their Social Security benefit status; however, we did not consider differences among minority groups. Yet minority group representation in the American population is growing. Between 1980 and 2000, both the Hispanic and black non-Hispanic shares of the population increased by 83% and 5%, respectively, while the white non-Hispanic share of the population decreased by 10% (Table 15 in U.S. Bureau of the Census, 2001). Census projects that by 2020 Hispanics will represent 17% of the population, blacks 13%, Native Americans 1%, and Asians 6%. Whites will represent only 64% of the population in 2020 compared with 80% in 1980 (Table 15 in U.S. Bureau of the Census, 2001).

In addition to their increasing presence, there are a number of other reasons to expect minority group differences in the economic well-being of future retirees. First, there are minority group differences in marital patterns. Among most age groups in the current population, we observe that white women are more likely than Hispanic and black women to ever marry. Black women who do marry are more likely than white and Hispanic women to divorce after the first marriage and they are least likely to ever remarry (Table 149 in U.S. Census Bureau, 2000). Second, there are minority group differences in educational attainment. The growth in educational attainment between 1970 and 2000 was greatest for black women, whose share completing high school more than doubled and whose share completing college more than tripled. Although by 2000 the gap in educational attainment between white and black women and white and Hispanic women had dramatically decreased, white women were still more likely than black and Hispanic women to complete high school and college (Table 216 in U.S. Census Bureau, 2001). Third, minority group differences are evident in work and earnings patterns. Although labor force participation rates of black women are higher than those for white and Hispanic women (Table 568 in U.S. Census Bureau, 2001), median weekly earnings among full-time workers are higher for white women than for black and Hispanic women (Table 621 in U.S. Census Bureau, 2001). Finally, minority group differences in economic well-being exist in the current retiree population. Among current female retirees, blacks are almost 2.5 times more likely to be poor and Hispanics are almost twice as likely to be poor as whites (Table 8.1 in Grad, 2002). We expect that many of the minority group differences in the current population will influence the retirement income and economic well-being of future retirees, and we expect the prospects for black and Hispanic women to be worse than those of white women.

In this paper we consider divorced women, an economically vulnerable group whose segment of the retiree population is expected to increase in the future, and compare the characteristics and retirement income of black non-Hispanics and Hispanics with those of white non-Hispanics–a topic seldom studied in the literature.[1] Our projections of the characteristics and income of the baby boom retiree population come from the Social Security Administration's (SSA) Modeling Income in the Near Term (MINT1).[2]

DESCRIPTION OF MINT

MINT is ideal for our analysis because it projects the characteristics and retirement income of future retirees; taking into account historical changes between and within birth cohorts in the level and distribution of earnings, labor force participation, educational attainment, marital patterns, and mortality across age, gender, and racial and ethnic groups.

For individuals born between 1926 and 1965, the MINT data system links their demographic information from the Census Bureau's 1990-93 Survey of Income and Program Participation (SIPP) panel data with their earnings histories from SSA administrative records. For our analysis, one of the most important features of MINT is that it includes lifetime marital histories and the characteristics of former and future spouses. Historical marital information is constructed in MINT using the SIPP–which provides detailed information on the first two and the most recent marriages–and the Panel Study of Income Dynamics (PSID)–which is used to impute the total number of marriages and marital changes occurring between the second and most recent marriage (Panis & Lillard, 1999). MINT projections of future marital changes are based on SIPP estimates using hazard analyses. Specifically, transitions into marriage and divorce are modeled using a gender specific continuous-time hazard model (Panis & Lillard, 1999).[3] Finally, once the number of former and future marriages and the timing of those marriages are estimated, the SIPP is used to identify the characteristics of spouses in those marriages.[4]

As well as information on earnings histories, marital histories, and the characteristics of future and former spouses, MINT includes independent projections of each retiree's entry to and exit from Social Security disability insurance (DI) rolls, age of first receipt of Social Security retirement benefits, and date of death. MINT also includes projected retirement income from private pensions, non-pension assets, earnings, and imputed rent from owner occupied housing. In addition, we use the marital history and earnings history information in MINT to compute Social Security benefits.

Thus, the MINT model directly measures the experiences of survey respondents, who represent different cohorts, up to the early 1990s and statistically projects their characteristics and income into the future, adjusting for expected demographic and socioeconomic changes. For these reasons, MINT is an ideal tool for gaining insight into the role that minority group status is expected to have on the economic well-being of women who are divorced at retirement.[5]

MARITAL STATUS OF RETIREES

We begin by examining the marital composition of future retirees and find that the MINT data system projects striking differences across minority groups (Table 1). Marriage is the most common marital state regardless of race or ethnicity; however, MINT data project that white women are significantly more likely than black and Hispanic women to be married at retirement. Only 40% of black women and 53% of Hispanic women are projected to be married at age 67. The corresponding estimate for white women is 57%. Divorce is also projected to be a common marital state at retirement. A quarter of all black women, 19% of white women, and 17% of Hispanic are projected to be divorced at retirement. It is these divorced women that we focus on in this paper. All subsequent tables and figures describe women who are projected to be divorced at age 67.

TABLE 1. Projected Marital Status of Women at Age 67, by Minority Group Status

Marital Status	White	Black	Hispanic
Divorced	19%	25%	17%
Never Married	5%	17%	8%
Married	57%	40%	53%
Widowed	18%	19%	22%
Total[a]	100%	100%	100%

[a]Due to rounding, totals may not sum to exactly 100%.
Source: Authors' calculations using MINT1 data.

DEMOGRAPHIC CHARACTERISTICS OF DIVORCED RETIREES

First we consider minority group differences in the demographic characteristics of divorced women at retirement (Table 2). We begin by examining the average age of Social Security take-up (retirement) across minority groups. Social Security benefit receipt before normal retirement age, thus early retirement, results in reduced annual benefits to account for the longer period over which benefits will be paid. Likewise, asset income that is annuitized at younger ages will result in lower

TABLE 2. Projected Demographic Characteristics of Divorced Women at Age 67, by Minority Group Status

	White		Black			Hispanic		
	Mean	Std. Dev.	Mean	Std. Dev.	Diff.[a]	Mean	Std. Dev.	Diff.[a]
Retirement Age	63.02	1.44	63.65	1.74	***	63.31	1.69	***
Marital History								
Age at First Marriage	22.23	5.07	23.44	6.36	***	22.53	4.91	NS
1 Marriage	0.60	0.49	0.70	0.46	***	0.69	0.46	***
2 Marriages	0.28	0.45	0.24	0.43	**	0.27	0.44	NS
3+ Marriages	0.12	0.33	0.06	0.23	***	0.05	0.21	***
Ever Had 10-Year Marriage	0.71	0.45	0.51	0.50	***	0.66	0.47	*
Education								
High School Dropout	0.05	0.22	0.12	0.33	***	0.22	0.41	***
High School Graduate	0.65	0.48	0.66	0.47	NS	0.61	0.49	NS
College Graduate	0.30	0.46	0.21	0.41	***	0.17	0.38	***
Renter	0.15	0.36	0.32	0.47	***	0.28	0.45	***
N of Cases (Unweighted)	2,195		266			189		

Notes:
NS = not signficant.
* = Significant at the 10% level.
** = Significant at the 5% level.
*** = Significant at the 1% level.
[a]T-test of significance of difference between the white and black/Hispanic statistics.
Source: Authors' calculations using MINT1 data.

annual payments. For these reasons we expect retirement age to be positively associated with retirement income. MINT data project that the average age of Social Security take-up will be between 63 and 64 for all minority groups. While significant differences across minority groups are projected, the differences are negligible. Black women are projected to delay Social Security benefit receipt the longest and white women are projected to retire the earliest.

There are also significant differences in marital histories across minority groups. Marital history, in combination with earnings history, is important for determining Social Security beneficiary status and benefit levels. The mean age that women first marry is between 22 and 23 for all minority groups. Given this young age, it's not surprising that a large number of divorced women married more than once before age 67. However, white women are more likely than black and Hispanic women to have multiple marriages (compare 40% for white women with 30% for black women and 32% for Hispanic women). These projections are similar to current statistics which show that black women are less likely than white and Hispanic women to remarry after divorce (Table 149 in U.S. Census Bureau, 2000). Finally, there are also significant differences in marriage duration across minority groups. White women are more likely than black and Hispanic women to have ever had a marriage last ten or more years. Seventy-one percent of white women, 66% of Hispanic women, and only 51% of black women have ever had a ten-year marriage. So while black women are more likely than white and Hispanic women to be divorced at retirement, they are less likely to be qualified for certain Social Security benefits because they don't meet the ten-year marriage requirement.[6]

Educational attainment in MINT represents, for the most part, the actual experiences of SIPP survey respondents in the early 1990s. For this reason, it's not surprising to find patterns of educational attainment among minority groups that are similar to those described earlier in this paper. In the MINT data system, white divorced women are less likely than black and Hispanic divorced women to not finish high school and they are more likely to complete college. Only 5% of white women in MINT do not have a high school education (compared with 12% of black women and 22% of Hispanic women). An additional 30% of white women, 21% of black women, and only 17% of Hispanic women have college degrees.

Finally, home ownership is considered an important asset in an individual's financial portfolio and thus is usually a positive indicator of an older person's total economic resources.[7] MINT projects large and significant differences across minority groups in home ownership. White women are half as likely as black and Hispanic women to be renters. Eighty-five percent of white women, 68% of black women, and 72% of Hispanic women are projected to own their homes at retirement.

BENEFICIARY STATUS OF DIVORCED RETIREES

Next we examine minority group differences in Social Security benefit status. Under Social Security program rules, divorced women may be eligible for retired-worker benefits and/or auxiliary benefits. To compute Social Security benefits, SSA first indexes annual earnings over a divorced woman's paid working career and then calculates her average indexed monthly earnings (AIME) and primary insurance amount (PIA)–the benefit payable at the normal retirement age.[8] Divorced women with 40 or more quarters of coverage (approximately 10 years of full-time work) over their work lives are considered fully insured and eligible for retired-worker benefits based on their own earnings history.

Some divorced women may also be entitled to auxiliary benefits if their former husbands are eligible for retired-worker benefits. Depending on whether her former husband is an ex-husband, deceased ex-husband, or deceased husband, a divorced woman is subject to different formulas for computing her auxiliary benefit and may or may not have to meet a ten-year marriage requirement. Although she describes herself as divorced, if eligible for an auxiliary benefit at retirement, a woman may receive Social Security benefits as a divorced spouse, surviving divorced spouse, or widow.[9]

Table 3 details the relationship between earnings and beneficiary status. For discussion purposes we separate out beneficiaries according to whether or not they meet the ten-year marriage requirement. We begin with divorced women who meet the ten-year marriage requirement. If a divorced woman has no earnings or too few quarters of coverage, then she has a PIA equal to zero and is ineligible for retired-worker benefits. Similarly, if her former husband has no earnings or too few quarters of coverage, then he has a PIA equal to zero (denoted as SPIA in Table 3). As a result, her former husband is also ineligible for retired-worker benefits and she is ineligible for auxiliary benefits based on his earnings history. In this case, she is considered a *nonbeneficiary*. An *auxiliary beneficiary* also has a PIA equal to zero; however, because her former husband has a positive PIA, she is entitled to a benefit based entirely on

TABLE 3. The Relationship Between Earnings and Social Security Benefit Status

Beneficiary Status	Comparison of Own and Spouse PIAs[a]	Approximate Size of Auxiliary Benefit	Final Benefit Based On	
			Own Earnings	Spouse Earnings
Met Ten-Year Marriage Requirement[b]				
Nonbeneficiary	PIA = 0, SPIA = 0	0	No	No
Auxiliary				
Divorced Spouse	PIA = 0, SPIA > 0	1/2 SPIA	No	Yes
Surviving Divorced Spouse	PIA = 0, SPIA > 0	SPIA	No	Yes
Widow	PIA = 0, SPIA > 0	SPIA	No	Yes
Dually Entitled				
Divorced Spouse	0 < PIA < 1/2 SPIA	1/2 SPIA - PIA	Yes	Yes
Surviving Divorced Spouse	0 < PIA < SPIA	SPIA - PIA	Yes	Yes
Widow	0 < PIA < SPIA	SPIA - PIA	Yes	Yes
Retired Worker[c]				
Divorced Spouse	PIA > 1/2 SPIA	0	Yes	No
Surviving Divorced Spouse	PIA > SPIA	0	Yes	No
Widow	PIA > SPIA	0	Yes	No
Did Not Meet Ten-Year Marriage Requirement				
Nonbeneficiary	PIA = 0	0	No	No
Retired Worker[c]				
Divorced Spouse	PIA > 0	0	Yes	No
Surviving Divorced Spouse	PIA > 0	0	Yes	No

Notes:

[a]PIA refers to a divorced woman's primary insurance amount and SPIA refers to her former husband's primary insurance amount. A PIA, the unreduced benefit that a retiree is eligible for, is computed by first indexing annual earnings over an individual's work life and then calculating the average indexed monthly earnings (AIME). The PIA is then computed directly from the AIME.

[b]Also includes those who don't have to meet the ten-year marriage requirement because their marriages ended in widowhood.

[c]For expository purposes only, we separated out retired workers into divorced spouses, surviving divorced spouses, and widows. However, SSA would classify all of these beneficiaries as retired workers.

her former husband's earnings history. A *dually entitled beneficiary* receives both a retired-worker and auxiliary benefit because her PIA is greater than zero, but less than her former husband's PIA. As a result, her benefit is based in part on her own earnings history and in part on her former husband's earnings history. Finally, a *retired-worker benefi-*

ciary is ineligible for auxiliary benefits because her PIA is greater than her former husband's PIA. Instead she receives a benefit based entirely on her own earnings history.

Next we discuss divorced women who did not meet the ten-year marriage requirement. In this case, how a divorced woman's PIA compares to her former husband's PIA is irrelevant because she is automatically ineligible for auxiliary benefits based on his earnings history. She can fall into only one of two beneficiary groups: a *nonbeneficiary* if her PIA is zero and a *retired-worker beneficiary* if her PIA is positive. Thus a divorced woman's Social Security beneficiary status depends on her marital history and earnings history, as well as the earnings histories of her former husbands.

Table 4 describes the projected beneficiary status of divorced women at age 67 by minority group status. The MINT data system projects that very few women will be ineligible for Social Security benefits at retirement. Hispanic women are four-times more likely than white women and twice as likely as black women to not qualify for benefits on their own or their former husbands' work histories. While less common today than in the past, some women do not qualify for benefits on their own. However, most have former husbands who do. Hispanic and black women are more likely than white women to be eligible for only auxiliary benefits as divorced spouses, surviving divorced spouses, or widows because they do not qualify for benefits on their own work histories (though they do qualify on their former husbands' work histories).[10]

TABLE 4. Projected Beneficiary Status of Divorced Women at Age 67, by Minority Group Status

	White		Black			Hispanic		
	Mean	Std. Dev.	Mean	Std. Dev.	Diff.*	Mean	Std. Dev.	Diff.*
Beneficiary Status								
Nonbeneficiary	0.01	0.12	0.02	0.12	NS	0.04	0.20	**
Auxiliary Beneficiary	0.03	0.18	0.07	0.25	***	0.06	0.24	*
Dually Entitled	0.36	0.48	0.17	0.37	***	0.28	0.45	***
Retired-Worker	0.60	0.49	0.75	0.43	***	0.62	0.48	NS

Notes:
NS = not signficant.
* = Significant at the 10% level.
** = Significant at the 5% level.
*** = Significant at the 1% level.
[a]T-test of significance of difference between the white and black/Hispanic statistics.
Source: Authors' calculations using MINT1 data.

Because of women's increased earnings and work patterns since the 1970s, most baby boom women are projected to be dually entitled or retired-worker beneficiaries at retirement and to receive benefits based in part or entirely on their own earnings histories. Dually entitled beneficiaries are those who: (1) have earnings histories that are lower than their former husband's earnings histories, *and* (2) have met the ten-year marriage requirement. Because their earnings tend to be more similar to their former husband's earnings and because they are less likely to meet the ten-year marriage requirement, it's not surprising that only 17% of black women are projected to be dually entitled beneficiaries at retirement (compared with 36% of white women and 28% of Hispanic women). Retired-worker beneficiaries, on the other hand, are those who: (1) have earnings histories that are similar to or higher than their former husband's earnings histories, *or* (2) have not met the ten-year marriage requirement. Overall, 60% of white women, 75% of black women, and 62% of Hispanic women are projected to be eligible for benefits on their own records and ineligible for auxiliary benefits. However, 45% of white women, 60% of black women, and 47% of Hispanic women are retired-worker beneficiaries solely because they failed to meet the ten-year marriage requirement (Figure 1). The majority of those who did not meet the ten-year marriage requirement (65% of white women, 60% of black women, and 56% of Hispanic women), would be eligible for auxiliary benefits as dually entitled beneficiaries and receive higher Social Security benefits if this requirement were eliminated.

Although most divorced women are projected to be retired-worker beneficiaries at retirement, many of them will become dually entitled surviving divorced spouses or widows and receive higher Social Security benefits when their former husbands die. This is because most divorced women have a PIA that is greater than one-half of their former husband's PIA, which makes them a retired-worker beneficiary while their former husband is alive, but less than 100% of their former husband's PIA, which makes them a dually entitled surviving divorced spouse or widow when their former husband dies. As Figure 2 shows, the majority of dually entitled beneficiaries will be surviving divorced spouses and widows (65% of white women, 80% of black women, and 76% of Hispanic women). Very few dually entitled beneficiaries will be divorced spouses.

FIGURE 1. Distibution of Projected Retired-Worker Benificiaries by Those With/Without Ten Years of Marriage and Minority Groups Status

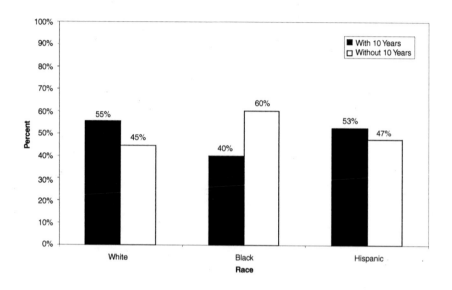

INCOME OF DIVORCED RETIREES

As already discussed, the majority of divorced women in all minority groups are projected to receive Social Security benefits at retirement. However, for most retirees, Social Security benefits represent only a portion of their overall retirement income. Most divorced women are projected to have additional sources of retirement income such as pension and asset income (Figure 3). MINT data project that more than half of all white and black women will have family pension income at retirement. In contrast, only 41% of Hispanic women are projected to have family pension income. A major difference across minority groups is in their ownership of assets. While 90% of white women are projected to have family asset income at retirement, only 77% of black women and 82% of Hispanic women will.

As we would expect, these differences have major consequences for the distribution of retirement income (Table 5).[11] Median retirement income is projected to be $18,385 (in 1998 dollars) for white women, but substantially less for black and Hispanic women (by 13% for black women and 34% for Hispanic women). MINT data also project more in-

FIGURE 2. Distribution of Projected Dually Entitled Beneficiaries, by Minority Group Status

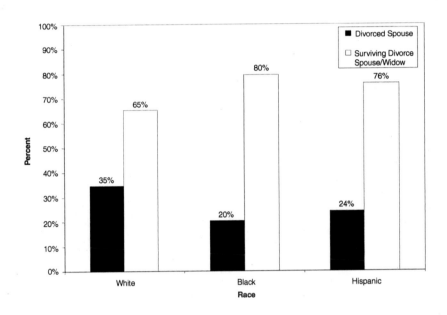

equality for black and Hispanic women than for white women–as can be seen by the 90/10 ratio. White women with income in the 90th percentile of the income distribution have 7.6 times more income than those with income in the 10th percentile of the income distribution. For black and Hispanic women, the comparable statistic is 9.9 times. Finally, not surprising is that black and Hispanic women have higher poverty rates at retirement than white women (compare 22.4% for black women and 29.3% for Hispanic women with only 12.4% for white women).

THE EFFECT OF DEMOGRAPHIC AND SOCIOECONOMIC CHARACTERISTICS ON INCOME

Next we consider the combined effect of the variables described above on retirement income. To do this we estimate a regression of the log of total income at age 67 by minority status. The results are presented in Table 6. Based on the descriptive analyses, the average divorced woman, regardless of minority status, retired at age 63, first

FIGURE 3. Projected Sources of Income for Divorced Women at Age 67, by Minority Group Status

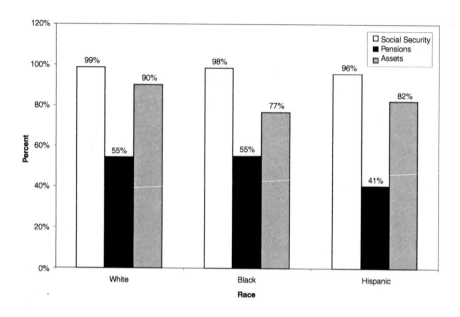

married at about age 22, married only once and was married for at least ten years, is high school educated, owns her home, is a retired-worker beneficiary, and has pension and asset income. Based on the regression results, a white woman fitting this description has $28,531 at retirement. A black woman fitting this description has only $25,594 at retirement. Finally, a Hispanic woman fitting this description has only $21,783 at retirement. The discussion below considers how deviations from the average or baseline case within minority groups influence retirement income.

Most of the variables have the expected direction of impact on retirement income. Delaying retirement, being a college graduate, and being a dually entitled surviving divorced spouse or widow are all associated with higher than average retirement income.[12] On the other hand, not having a high school degree, renting, being a nonbeneficiary, auxiliary beneficiary, dually entitled spouse, or retired-worker beneficiary without ten years of marriage, and not having pension or asset income are all associated with lower than average retirement income.[13]

TABLE 5. Distribution of Income of Divorced Women at Age 67, by Minority Group Status ($1,998)

	White	Black	Hispanic
Mean	$25,998	$21,030	$18,308
Median	$18,385	$16,062	$12,191
10th Percentile	$7,265	$4,673	$4,251
90th Percentile	$55,210	$46,470	$42,201
90/10 Ratio	7.6	9.9	9.9
Poverty Rate	12.4	22.4	29.3

Source: Authors' calculations using MINT1 data.

Many of the variables in the regression equations for white and Hispanic women have a significant impact on retirement income, while much fewer in the regression equation for black women do. It turns out that for all minority groups a divorced woman's marital history has relatively little impact on her income at retirement. However, some of this effect might be captured in the beneficiary status variables which also reflect her marital history.

Although many variables are important predictors of retirement income in the individual regression equations, very few have a significantly different impact on retirement income between whites and blacks or whites and Hispanics. A divorced woman's age at first marriage, dual entitlement to surviving divorced spouse or widow benefits, and rights to pension and asset income all have a significantly different impact on the retirement incomes of whites and blacks. White women who are dually entitled surviving divorced spouses or widows have 8% more ($e^{.079} - 1$) income at retirement than retired-worker beneficiaries. The comparable estimate for black women is almost 6 times higher–45% ($e^{.374} - 1$). Rights to pension and asset income also have a significantly different impact on the retirement incomes of white and black women. Divorced women without pensions have retirement income that is 45% less for whites and 50% less for blacks than their counterparts with pensions. The minority group differences are more dramatic for asset income. Asset ownership has a much larger impact on white divorced women–whose retirement income is 26% less than the average if they don't have assets–than on black divorced women–whose retirement income is only 3% less than the average if they don't have assets.

TABLE 6. Regression Results of Log Income of Divorced Women at Age 67, by Minority Group Status

	White		Black			Hispanic		
	Coeff.	Std. Err.	Coeff.	Std. Err.	Diff.[a]	Coeff.	Std. Err.	Diff.[a]
Retirement Age	3.526***	0.843	3.517	2.339	NS	6.813***	2.608	NS
Retirement Age Squared	−0.027***	0.007	−0.027	0.018	NS	−0.053***	0.020	NS
Marital History								
Age at First Marriage	0.027	.018	−0.055	0.044	*	−0.120**	0.056	**
Age at First Marriage Squared	0.000	0.000	0.001	0.001	NS	0.002**	0.001	**
2 Marriages	−0.020	0.038	−0.161	0.115	NS	0.092	0.108	NS
3+ Marriages	0.141**	0.056	−0.028	0.170	NS	0.016	0.257	NS
Education								
High School Dropout	−0.478***	0.097	−0.330**	0.157	NS	−0.236**	0.104	*
College Graduate	0.293***	0.035	0.180	0.135	NS	0.453***	0.140	NS
Renter	−0.221***	0.046	−0.185*	0.096	NS	−0.378***	0.102	NS
Beneficiary Status								
Nonbeneficiary	−2.654***	0.417	−2.345***	0.191	NS	−1.733***	0.243	*
Auxiliary Beneficiary	−0.193**	0.093	−0.050	0.220	NS	−0.423**	0.202	NS
Dually Entitled	0.079**	0.039	0.374***	0.110	**	0.287**	0.135	NS
Dually Entitled*Ex-Spouse	−0.495***	0.048	−0.702***	0.202	NS	−0.762***	0.200	NS
Retired Worker*No Ten-Year Marriage	−0.137***	0.043	−0.118	0.110	NS	−0.041	0.132	NS
No Pension Income	−0.592***	0.035	−0.792***	0.097	*	−0.550***	0.111	NS
No Asset Income	−0.296***	0.052	−0.029	0.109	**	−0.351***	0.114	NS
Constant	−104.101***	27.046	−101.846	75.221	NS	−207.804**	83.793	NS
R-Squared	0.426		0.458			0.575		

Notes:
NS = not significant.
* = Significant at the 10% level.
** = Significant at the 5% level.
*** = Significant at the 1% level.
[a]T-test of significance of difference between the white and black/Hispanic models.
Source: Authors' calculations using MINT1 data.

A divorced woman's age at first marriage, educational attainment, and nonbeneficiary status all have a significantly different impact on the retirement incomes of whites and Hispanics. White women without high school degrees have 38% less income than those with high school degrees, while Hispanic women without high school degrees have only 21% less income than those with high school degrees. The difference in incomes between nonbeneficiaries and retired worker beneficiaries is also larger for white women than for Hispanic women (compare 93% for white women with only 82% for Hispanic women).

ACCOUNTING FOR THE MINORITY GAP IN TOTAL INCOME

To understand how important the factors described above are in accounting for the minority gap in total income, we decomposed the gap using the means and coefficients from the regression. To do this we consider what black and Hispanic women would look like if they had the characteristics or returns to characteristics that white women do. Table 7 reports the size of the gap, as well as the shares of the gap ex-

TABLE 7. Decomposition of Gap in Total Income at Age 67, by Minority Group Status

	Black		Hispanic	
	Log	Dollars	Log	Dollars
White Income	9.827	25,998	9.827	25,998
Black/Hispanic Income	9.590	21,030	9.400	18,308
Gap in Income	0.237	4,968	0.427	7,689
Decomposition of Gap:				
Differences in Characteristics	41%	2,037	70%	5,382
Age at Retirement	−1%	−50	1%	77
Marital History	−1%	−50	3%	231
Education	16%	795	22%	1,692
Renter	13%	646	11%	846
Beneficiary Status	14%	696	9%	692
Have No Pension Income	−2%	−99	18%	1,384
Have No Asset Income	2%	99	6%	461
Differences in Returns to Characteristics	49%	2,434	26%	1,999
Joint Interaction of Differences	10%	497	4%	308
Total	100%	4,968	100%	7,689

Source: Authors' calculations using MINT1 data.

plained by three components: differences in characteristics, differences in returns to characteristics, and the joint interaction of differences. This last component can be interpreted as the effect of characteristics and returns to characteristics beyond their individual effects.

The income gap between whites and blacks is .237 in log income or $4,968. Differences in characteristics between the groups account for 41% of the gap, while differences in returns to characteristics account for 49% of the gap. Ten percent of the gap is explained by the joint interaction of the differences. Differences in education levels account for 16% or $795 of the gap in income.[14] Also important in explaining the minority gap are differences in beneficiary status (14%) and differences in home ownership (13%).

The income gap between whites and Hispanics is .427 in log income or $7,689. Differences in characteristics between the groups account for 70% of the gap. Differences in returns to characteristics, however, account for only 26% of the gap. Four percent of the gap is explained by the joint interaction of the differences. As with black women, differences in education levels explain most of the minority gap in income between white and Hispanic women (22% or $1,692).[15] Differences in pension receipt account for another 18% or $1,384 of the gap, and home ownership accounts for 11% or $846 of the gap. Differences in beneficiary status account for only 9% or $692 of the gap.

CONCLUSION

Recent trends suggest that minority groups and divorced women will represent a much larger segment of the future retiree population. Historically, these two groups have experienced double-digit poverty rates in retirement. For these reasons, we expect an increase in the proportion of economically vulnerable aged women when the baby boom cohort retires.

Using a unique data source on the income and characteristics of future retirees, we examined the impact of minority status on the economic well-being of divorced women in the baby boom cohort. We found large minority group differences in the retirement income of future divorced women. White women are projected to be the best off in retirement, while Hispanic women are projected to be the worst off. Our results indicate that these differences are driven largely by differences in characteristics across minority groups. Only a few of the variables that we tested had a differential impact on the retirement income of white, black, and Hispanic women, suggesting that differences in returns to characteristics explain little of the differences in retirement income. That is, being college educated, owning a home, and having pension and asset income, for example, are associated with increased retirement income for all racial and ethnic groups. However, because black and Hispanic women are less likely than white women to be college educated, to own their home, and to have pension and asset income, their retirement income tends to be lower than that of white women.

Policy options to address the retirement needs of divorced women are seldom discussed. Clearly some women would benefit from the elimination of the ten-year marriage requirement. In addition, most women would benefit from a policy that increases the auxiliary benefit that divorced spouses are entitled to based on their former husband's earnings record. Similar proposals are currently being heard for widow beneficiaries. Many of these women might also benefit from increased income targeted at the elderly through the Supplemental Security Income (SSI) program. This could be accomplished by increasing the benefits and/or income and resource limits. Because this program is designed to ensure that the neediest elderly receive SSI benefits, it requires individuals to meet certain income and resource limits. While benefits have been increased over the years to keep up with inflation, the income and resource limits have not. Consequently, over time the elderly have been increasingly more likely to be ineligible for SSI benefits. Finally, another policy option might be to institute minimum Social Security benefits. However, this proposition is less promising because there is no basis for identifying economically vulnerable aged beneficiaries on SSA administrative earnings records.

The Social Security Trustees' report projects rising earnings in future years with adequate productivity and limited inflation (Table V.B1 in U.S. Board of Trustees of the Federal Old-Age and Survivors Insurance and Disability Insurance Trust Funds, 2002). Based on our analysis, however, a rising tide will not lift all boats; there will still be segments of the baby boom retired population that are economically vulnerable. While this finding is consistent with a number of previous research studies, our analysis is one of the first to shed light on what to expect for divorced women of different racial and ethnic groups.[16]

NOTES

1. Among current retirees, the poverty rates of never married women are also very high; however, this group represents such a small proportion of the female retiree population that it isn't statistically feasible to analyze minority group differences. For this reason we focus only on divorced female retirees in this paper.

2. SSA's Office of Policy developed the MINT data system with substantial assistance from the Brookings Institution, the RAND Corporation, and the Urban Institute (Panis & Lillard, 1999; Toder, Uccello, O'Hare, Favreault, Ratcliffe, Smith et al., 1999; Butrica, Iams, Moore, & Waid, 2001). A new version of MINT–known as MINT3–is currently being completed by the Urban Institute and the Brookings Institution (although MINT2 exists, it was created for internal use within SSA until MINT3 was completed). A preliminary version of MINT3 suggests that overall poverty rates will be lower than in MINT1. Despite this difference, we expect the relationships described in this paper to remain the same using MINT3.

3. The regressors in the marriage hazard are age, number of years unmarried, number of marriages, race, education, whether the individual was ever widowed, and permanent income. The regressors in the divorce hazard are age, marriage duration, number of marriages, education, race, and an indicator for pre- and post-1980 calendar year. The latter variables identify the year that divorce rates stabilized at a relatively high level (Goldstein, 1999). These models were developed on the 1990 and 1991 SIPP panels and found to be a good fit when tested on the 1992 and 1993 SIPP panels.

4. This procedure involves two steps. The first step is to impute the birth date, race, Hispanic ethnicity, education, disability status, and date of disability onset of spouses who were never part of the SIPP panels. The imputation algorithms are based on empirical couple distributions in the SIPP data (Panis & Lillard, 1999). The second step is to use a statistical matching algorithm to identify actual spouses in the MINT data system with similar characteristics to those statistically imputed (Toder, Uccello, O'Hare, Favreault, Ratcliffe, Smith et al., 1999).

5. Our analysis focuses on baby boomers who were born between 1946 and 1960. We omit those born 1961-1964 from the analysis because with fewer years of observed data we are less confident in their projections of retirement income. Because we estimate the impact of characteristics on the log of total income, we also include only those with non-zero retirement income (this represents nearly 100% of white, 99% of black, and 97% of Hispanic female divorced retirees). Finally, we exclude those who are projected to receive DI benefits.

6. An old-age Social Security benefit reflects an individual's earnings history, as well as his/her marital history. As such, eligibility for certain Social Security benefits requires that the marriage connected with the paid benefit last at least ten years before divorce. Social Security program rules are discussed in more detail in the next section.

7. The opposite is true for older people who are "house-rich and cash-poor." However, financial instruments are available to help these people derive income from the value of their homes.

8. Currently the normal retirement age is 65. For the baby boom cohorts in our analysis, it is scheduled to increase gradually from age 66 for those born in 1946 to age 67 for those born in 1960.

9. Some divorced women may actually receive widow benefits at retirement if the widow benefit, from a previous marriage that ended in widowhood, is larger than the divorced spouse or surviving divorced spouse benefit, from a previous marriage that ended in divorce. As a result, the type of Social Security benefit that a woman receives may not reflect her self-described marital status (Butrica & Iams, 2000).

10. This result might seem counterintuitive because current statistics show that black women are more likely to work than white and Hispanic women (Table 568 in U.S. Census Bureau, 2001); however, it may be that their work history is more sporadic and makes them more likely than white women to have too few quarters of coverage or too little earnings to qualify for their own benefits.

11. Our measure of total income comprises Social Security benefits, earnings, assets, and pensions. Income flows from assets are annuitized using a multivariate annuity calculator that accounts for age, gender, education, and race.

12. We included an interaction term (dually entitled*ex-spouse) to capture the differential impact that being a dually entitled divorced spouse or dually entitled surviving divorced spouse or widow has on retirement income. The interaction term is negative and significant for all minority groups, suggesting that dually entitled ex-spouses have less income at retirement than dually entitled surviving divorced spouses and widows. This result is not surprising given that, for identical earnings, the Social Security benefit formula provides a surviving divorced spouse or widow with twice the auxiliary benefit amount it provides a divorced spouse.

13. We also included an interaction term (retired worker*no ten-year marriage) to capture the differential impact that being a retired-worker beneficiary with and without ten years of marriage has on retirement income. The interaction term is negative which implies that those who are retired-worker beneficiaries because they failed to meet the ten-year marriage requirement have less income at retirement than all other retired-worker beneficiaries. This result is not surprising since, as we already discussed, most retired workers without ten years of marriage would be eligible for auxiliary benefits as dually entitled beneficiaries and receive higher Social Security benefits if this requirement were eliminated. This variable was significant only for white women. It had no significant impact on the retirement income of black women, despite the large proportion who are projected to be retired-worker beneficiaries without ten years of marriage (Figure 1).

14. Although not shown, the differences in returns to education explain only 2% of the minority gap in income between white and black women.

15. If Hispanic women had the same returns to education as white women, the minority gap in income would increase not decrease as in the case for black women. This is because the returns to education are actually higher for Hispanic women than they are for white women.

16. A number of studies (Easterlin, MacDonald, & Macunovich, 1990; Easterlin, Schaeffer, & Macunovich, 1993; Sabelhaus & Manchester, 1995; Keister, 2000) conclude that most baby boomers will enjoy higher incomes and wealth in retirement than their parents did, but that some subgroups, such as nonmarried women and less educated persons, will fall behind.

REFERENCES

Ahlburg, D. A., & De Vita C. J. (1992). New realities of the American family. *Population Bulletin 47*, 1-44.

Butrica, B. A., & Iams, H. M. (2000). Divorced women at retirement: Projections of economic well-being in the near future. *Social Security Bulletin 63*(3), 3-12.

Butrica, B. A., Iams, H. M., Moore, J. H., & Waid, M. D. (2001). *Methods in modeling income in the near term (MINT1)* (ORES Working Paper Series No. 91). Washington, DC: Social Security Administration, Office of Policy.

DaVanzo, J., & Rahman, M. O. (1993). American families: Trends and correlates. *Population Index 59*(3), 350-386.

Easterlin, R. A., MacDonald, C., & Macunovich, D. J. (1990). Retirement prospects of the baby boom generation: A different perspective. *The Gerontologist 30*(6), 776-783.

Easterlin, R. A., Schaeffer, C. M., & Macunovich, D. J. (1993). Will the baby boomers be less well off than their parents? Income, wealth, and family circumstances over the life cycle in the United States. *Population and Development Review 19*(3), 497-522.

Goldstein, J. R. (1999). The leveling of divorce in the United States. *Demography 36*(3), 409-414.

Grad, S. (2002). *Income of the population 55 or older, 2000* (SSA Publication No. 13-11871). Washington, DC: U.S. Government Printing Office.

Keister, L. A. (2000). *Wealth in America: Trends in wealth inequality.* New York: Cambridge University Press.

Norton, A. J., & Miller, L. F. (1992). Marriage, divorce, and remarriage in the 1990's. *Current Population Reports: Special Studies* (Series P-23 No. 180). Washington, DC: Bureau of the Census.

Panis, C., & Lillard, L. (1999). *Near term model development* (Final Report. SSA Contract No: 600-96-27335). Santa Monica, CA: RAND.

Sabelhaus, J., & Manchester, J. (1995). Baby boomers and their parents: How does their economic well-being compare in middle age? *Journal of Human Resources 30*(4), 791-806.

Toder, E., Uccello, C., O'Hare, J., Favreault, M., Ratcliffe, C., Smith, K. et al. (1999). *Modeling income in the near term-projections of retirement income through 2020 for the 1931-1960 birth cohorts* (Final Report. SSA Contract No: 600-96-27332). Washington, DC: The Urban Institute.

U.S. Board of Trustees of the Federal Old-Age and Survivors Insurance and Disability Insurance Trust Funds. (2002). *Annual report.* Washington, DC: U.S. Government Printing Office.

U.S. Bureau of the Census. (2001). *Statistical abstract of the United States: 2001 (121st edition).* Washington, DC: U.S. Bureau of the Census.

U.S. Bureau of the Census. (2000). *Statistical abstract of the United States: 2000 (120th edition).* Washington, DC: U.S. Bureau of the Census.

Gender, Widowhood, and Long-Term Care in the Older Mexican American Population

Jacqueline L. Angel, PhD
Nora Douglas
Ronald J. Angel, PhD

SUMMARY. The objective of this study is to examine the influences of gender on long-term care service use among older Mexican American widows and widowers. Our analysis is based on a sample of 773 widows and 183 widowers from the Longitudinal Study of Elderly Mexican American Health (H-EPESE). In this sample widows resemble widowers in terms of demographic and health characteristics. However, widows report more financial strain than widowers and a greater welfare dependency (SSI) and Medicaid use. Among those who suffered diminished health, widows were more likely than widowers to use community-based long-term care services whereas widowers were more likely

---

Address correspondence to: Jacqueline L. Angel, Center on Health and Social Policy, P.O. Box Y, The University of Texas at Austin, Austin TX 78713 (E-mail: jangel@mail.utexas.edu).

This study is supported, in part, by a grant from the National Institute on Aging (NIA) (1R01 AG10939-03) with supplementary funding from the LBJ School Policy Research Institute Urban Issues Program.

An earlier version of this paper was presented at the American Sociological Association meeting, Chicago, Illinois, August 18, 2002.

[Haworth co-indexing entry note]: "Gender, Widowhood, and Long-Term Care in the Older Mexican American Population." Angel, Jacqueline L., Nora Douglas, and Ronald J. Angel. Co-published simultaneously in *Journal of Women & Aging* (The Haworth Press, Inc.) Vol. 15, No. 2/3, 2003, pp. 89-105; and: *Widows and Divorcees in Later Life: On Their Own Again* (ed: Carol L. Jenkins) The Haworth Press, Inc., 2003, pp. 89-105. Single or multiple copies of this article are available for a fee from The Haworth Document Delivery Service [1-800-HAWORTH, 9:00 a.m. - 5:00 p.m. (EST). E-mail address: docdelivery@haworthpress.com].

10.1300/J074v15n02_06

to enter a nursing home. Widows also had more instrumental and socioemotional support than widowers. Serious cognitive and functional impairment, though, places widows and widowers at the same risk of institutionalization. We end with a discussion of the policy implications of these findings. *[Article copies available for a fee from The Haworth Document Delivery Service: 1-800-HAWORTH. E-mail address: <docdelivery@haworthpress.com> Website: <http://www.HaworthPress.com> © 2003 by The Haworth Press, Inc. All rights reserved.]*

KEYWORDS. Long-term care, Mexican American, widows, widowers, Medicaid use, nursing home

INTRODUCTION

One of the most difficult transitions in later life is the loss of a life-long companion. Because of women's longer life spans and the fact that they tend to marry men who are older than themselves, widows outnumber widowers by over four times, 10.0 million to 2.5 million in 2000 (Fields and Casper, 2001). Even though the loss of a spouse is a normal life course transition, it can have serious negative emotional consequences, especially for women. Researchers have documented a decrease in general well-being and an increase in depression associated with widowhood (Barrett, 2000; Carr, House, and Kessler, 2000; Lynam, 1985; Umberson, Wortman, and Kessler, 1992).

Yet the loss of a spouse has far more than emotional consequences; it has potentially serious practical implications. Once she has lost her husband an older widow can suffer a substantial drop in income, placing her at elevated risk of poverty (Holden and Smock, 1991; Hurd and Wise, 1989), and possibly, of poor health (Fitzpatrick and Entmacher, 2000). More than half of elderly widows living in poverty were not poor before the death of their husbands. One study revealed that within three years of the death of her husband, a widow's income drops by 44 percent on average (Holden and Kuo, 1996). For couples with modest incomes, a drop of this magnitude greatly increases the risk of poverty for the surviving partner (Zick and Smith, 1991). Given the lower average incomes of blacks and Hispanics at all ages, Hispanic widows are at particularly high risk, and those who live alone experience the highest poverty rates (38.3 percent) of all racial and ethnic groups (U.S. Bureau of the Census, 2001).

The economically disadvantaged Hispanic widows face results from a combination of two systematic risks, the first results from the gender-based earnings disadvantages that women face across the life course, and the second from the generally depressed earnings capacity of Hispanics as a group. Middle-class, educated women today are far more conscious of their own financial situations than were their mothers or grandmothers. In previous generations a widow's situation largely depended upon the arrangements her husband made for their joint retirement and for her welfare when he was gone. A woman with substantial property and the income from resources acquired by her husband while he was alive was in far better financial condition in old age than a woman whose husband left her with little. Such a situation placed different groups of women at very different risks of poverty in old age. Although the situation may have improved for middle-class women, for poor women it remains largely the same. Depressed asset accumulation opportunities over a couple's life course leave the widow to suffer the more serious consequences at the end of life. In order to understand the situation of widows, therefore, it is necessary to examine various groups differently.

It is particularly important to take specific characteristics associated with an increased risk of poverty in old age into account. As we have noted, one serious dimension of economic disadvantage in the United States is associated with race and Hispanic ethnicity. Older single Hispanics often have very few resources to carry them through the later years of life and are consequently at extremely high risk of dependency. Sixty-one percent of elderly Hispanics depend on Social Security alone because they have no private retirement income while fewer than half of elderly non-Hispanic whites have no private retirement plan. In addition, 25 percent of older Hispanics rely on Supplemental Security Income, while only 5 percent of non-Hispanic whites rely on this needs-based program (Angel and Angel, 1997). Although non-Hispanic whites earn on average about fifty to sixty percent more than Mexican Americans, non-Hispanic whites have on average ten times more material wealth in the form of assets than Mexican Americans (Angel and Angel, 1996). Assets are a major source of economic security for widows so the drastically lower level of asset accumulation over the life course among blacks and Hispanics has serious implications for women in later life.

BACKGROUND

In this analysis we focus on older Mexican-origin widows, largely because of their seriously elevated risk of poverty (Angel and Angel, 1998). We focus on Mexican-origin widows for two other reasons as well. First, Hispanics are quickly becoming the largest American minority group in the United States, with the number over 65 projected to grow from 2.5 million in 2000 to 13 million by 2050. Among Hispanics, those of Mexican origin make up the largest number (Angel and Angel, 1998). Second, one-quarter of this older Hispanic population will be 80 or over by 2030, an age range in which the risk of dependency increases greatly (Anderton, Barrett, and Bogue, 1997).

Specific characteristics of the Mexican-origin population have potentially important implications for widows. Higher fertility among the Mexican-origin population provides greater opportunities for older parents to live with or close to their children, potentially reducing the risk of institutionalization (Angel, Angel, and Markides, 2000). The ways in which the poor, and Mexican Americans in particular, deal with poverty and poor health has been the source of much speculation. It has been suggested that the familistic orientation that has often been used to characterize traditional Mexican culture may represent a mechanism for dealing with poverty (Angel and Tienda, 1982). Mexican Americans are more likely to live with others, either a spouse or with their family, than non-Hispanic whites (Lee and Angel, 2002), and certain evidence suggests that among Hispanics a norm of caring for family members increases the probability that an elderly parent who is in poor health will be cared for at home (Wallace, Levy-Storms, and Ferguson, 1995).

Cultural norms that place responsibility for aging parents with adult children increase the possibility that older widowed Mexican-origin individuals will live with one of their children. The economic vulnerability of older Hispanic women and the fact that the family may be less able to provide informal support in the years to come, though, leads us to ask two policy relevant questions, the first whether or not social support prevents institutionalization for older Mexican-origin individuals at all, and the second whether providing more formal community care might supplement that provided by the family and allow widows to remain in the community rather than enter a nursing home in the event of serious incapacity.

Although the literature on social support and health consistently demonstrates that individuals with adequate social support are at lower risk of institutionalization than those with inadequate social support

(Wolf, Freedman, and Soldo, 1997), what is less clear is the degree to which these findings are applicable to frail and disabled Mexican-origin widows. Little evidence exists, although investigators who have examined the predictors of home health care use among elderly Hispanics have found that disabled Hispanics have a higher probability of using paid home health care when their children live nearby (Wallace, Campbell, and Lew Ting, 1994). In addition, adult daughters tend to provide more household and personal care to disabled Hispanic parents than is the case for non-Hispanic whites, and they tend to express a need for and use more in-home services and adult day care when it is available (Wallace and Lew-Ting, 1992). These findings raise the possibility that informal resources may act as a substitute for nursing home care, especially for adult daughters of Mexican-origin widows who provide them with considerable resources to stay in the community with compromised health.

When one deals with the Mexican-origin population, it is impossible to ignore issues related to place of birth and age of migration. Nativity plays a significant role in determining patterns of access to and reliance upon social support (Angel, Angel, McClelland, and Markides, 1996). Data from the 1988 National Survey of Hispanic Elderly People indicate that the difficulties associated with immigration late in life, such as language proficiency and retirement security, may undermine an older person's morale or general sense of personal control and interfere with the ability to perform instrumental activities of daily living (Angel and Angel, 1992).

In this paper we examine the association between widowhood and several other factors, including income, social support, and long-term care service use among widowed elderly Mexican Americans over an eight-year period. Our objective is to answer the two questions we raised earlier, (1) whether the availability of social support reduces the risk of institutionalization among older Mexican-origin widows, and (2) the extent of community care they employ. We begin by documenting several risk factors for institutionalization.

We expect that several background variables, including age at migration, strongly influence differentiated patterns of informal support for widowed men and for women, and affect the propensity to use community care as an alternative to nursing facilities. Because the loss of a spouse requires that a person reorient and restructure his or her local support network (Ferraro, 1984; Utz, Carr, Nesse, and Wortman, 2002), we hypothesize that widows will be more likely to live with their children than widowers and will, therefore, be less likely to use nursing homes. We expect to show that while poor health increases the general risk of entering the nursing home, that risk is conditioned by the availability of social support. Because Hispanics have larger families and theoretically greater access to social support than non-Hispanic whites, we expect that they will have a greater tendency to remain in the community and to use community-based services than non-Hispanic elderly. Following this same logic, we expect widowers to be less likely than widows to rely on family in the event of poor health and be more likely to enter a nursing home.

DATA AND METHODS

We employ the Longitudinal Survey of Mexican American Elderly Health (Hispanic Established Populations for Epidemiological Studies of the Elderly, H-EPESE) which is a large, multistage probability sample of Mexican American elderly who reside in the five southwestern states of Texas, California, New Mexico, Arizona, and Colorado. The survey consisted of a sample of 3,050 individuals 65 and over interviewed in 1993-1994. Information from a knowledgeable proxy was obtained for individuals who were unable to complete the entire interview themselves because of infirmity or cognitive incapacity. The original panel was re-contacted three more times, in 1994/1995 and again in 1998/1999 and 2000/01. The H-EPESE sample of widows (n = 956) resembles the nation's widowed elderly populations. In 1994, among Mexican Americans 65 and over in the United States, 18.0 percent were widowed men and 41.2 percent were widowed women. In the H-EPESE sample, representing the Hispanic population 65 and over in the Southwest, 14.2 percent of the men and 43.9 percent of the women reported they were widows, reflecting the Census Bureau's estimates of the total number of Latino elderly widows in the United States.

Measures

Independent variables. The survey includes basic demographic information at baseline, including age (categorized as 65-69 versus 70-79, 80 and over), gender, education, living arrangements (alone versus head of household, non-head of household), nativity (born in Mexico versus United States), age at migration (came to the United States at age 50 or beyond versus native or younger age), and acculturation (Spanish language of interview versus English language). Information is also available on the economic situation of the household: poverty threshold, health insurance coverage, assets (housing and cash), and perceived financial strain. Financial strain was based on responses to two questions: The first question was: "How much difficulty do you have in meeting monthly payments on your bills?" Those who reported any difficulty were scored 1. The second question was "At the end of the month, do you usually end up with some money left over, just enough to make ends meet, or not enough money to make ends meet?" Those who reported that they did not have enough money to make ends meet were scored 1. For each individual, we created a new financial strain variable that is scored 1 if any of each of these variables is 1, and 0 otherwise.

Non-economic resources include measures of the amount of instrumental and socioemotional supports received. Instrumental support is measured by three responses to the question: "Can you count on your children in times of trouble most of the time, some of the time, or rarely?" Socioemotional support was based on frequency of church attendance: often (weekly/monthly), sometimes (a few times a year) or never or almost never.

Mental health and functioning consisted of several domains of cognitive and physical disability. Each follow-up includes detailed self-reports of health and functioning measure limitations with basic activities of daily living, cognitive impairment, and depression (CES-D). Limitation in activities of daily living is dichotomized to indicate whether the respondent reported at least some limitation in personal care (bathing, grooming, dressing, walking, transferring, eating, and toileting). In order to control for psychological and cognitive functioning we include the Mini Mental Status Exam (MMSE) and the Center for Epidemiologic Studies Depression Scale (CES-D). The MMSE is based on the correct responses to a standard battery of memory and reasoning items. A score 18-23 indicates mild cognitive impairment, and scores below 18 were coded as severely impaired. The CES-D captures different levels of depressive affect (a score of 16 or higher indicates chronic depression).

Dependent variables. Long-term care service use was defined as home- and community-based services and nursing facilities. *Community-based services* refer to transportation for the elderly, senior center/church, adult day care, and home delivered meals. *Home health care* refers to personal assistance (service that assists with such tasks as dressing, grooming or household chores), visiting nurse, nurses' aide, physical therapist and use of an emergency response service. *Any senior service* refers to community care service and/or home health care utilization, plus receipt of food stamps. *Nursing facility use* was defined in terms of ever having been institutionalized (including custodial, rehabilitative, and skilled nursing facility).

RESULTS

Table 1 presents the respondent status and the vital status of the respondents at the four waves of the survey separately for widows (n = 773) and widowers (n = 183). By the second interview, 15.3 percent of the original widowers had died compared to 6.9 percent of widows. More than 10 percent (14.2 percent) of widowers and 11.4 percent of widows refused to participate either because they were institutionalized, were too ill to be interviewed, or they had moved to Mexico where they could not be recontacted. By the third interview, approximately one-third (34.4 percent) of the widower respondents had died, and 13.7 percent had entered a nursing home, or been lost to follow-up. One-fifth of the widows had died by time three and 13.9 percent were loss to follow-up. At the final interview, almost half of the widowers had died (46.5 percent) versus 29.6 percent for widows. Almost one-half of the widows and about one-third of widowers were re-interviewed, and slightly more than 13 percent of the widowed sample did not respond at the fourth wave of the survey.

TABLE 1. Respondent Status at Four Waves

Respondent Status	Time one 1993-94		Time two 1995-96		Time three 1998-99		Time four 2000-01	
	Widower	Widow	Widower	Widow	Widower	Widow	Widower	Widow
Self	83.6	88.4	57.4	71.7	39.3	54.9	29.5	47.2
Assisted Proxy	7.7	5.7	6.0	5.4	2.7	2.7	3.3	2.6
Proxy Only	8.7	6.0	7.1	4.7	9.8	8.3	6.6	6.7
Dead	Na	Na	15.3	6.9	34.4	20.3	46.5	29.6
Refused	Na	Na	3.8	2.7	2.2	4.3	2.2	4.9
Unknown	Na	Na	10.4	8.7	11.5	9.6	12.0	8.9
Total	(183)	(773)	(183)	(773)	(183)	(773)	(183)	(773)

Source: Longitudinal Study of Elderly Mexican American Health (1993 – 2001)

Next, the analysis compares the demographic background, economic situation, characteristics and relative physical and cognitive capacities for widowers and widows across the eight years. Using all four waves of the panel allows us to document the prevalence of economic and health vulnerabilities in a large sample of Mexican American elderly men and women who are at high risk of dependency on others for formal supports due to the death of a spouse. The table also presents social and health care utilization analyses of the widows by gender. As Table 2 reveals, very few demographic characteristics distinguish between the widows and the widowers. Overall, widows and widowers report similar levels of health and functional limitations. There are a few exceptions with respect to economic situation: widows were less structurally incorporated into the United States, i.e., they were more likely than widowers to report welfare assistance (food stamps and Medicaid), to report less retirement income, and to experience more financial strain.

The table also demonstrates significant differences in health care utilization patterns for men and for women. Widows were more likely than widowers to use any type of senior service, home care, or home health care service. Conversely, widowers were more likely than widows to have used a nursing home.

Finally, the table shows that widows were more likely than widowers to receive a great deal of instrumental support and to draw a great comfort from attendance at places of worship.

In Table 3 we predict the community care utilization consequences of widowhood. The analyses assess the extent to which community-based care service use is a function of gender and widowhood. Each type of home and community care service is coded as a binomial dependent variable, and demographic, economic, social support, and functional health status variables appear on the right hand side of the equation. The main independent variable, "widowed females," is coded 1 for widows and 0 for widowers (reference category).

The multivariate results indicate several key significant predictors of community care use. In all three models, when other health-related factors are taken into account, widows are more likely than widowers to use all types of community-based long-term care services. Individuals who reported higher levels of psychological well-being were also more likely than those without serious disabling depression to use home health care. Conversely, late life migrants are less likely than native born and early migrants to use any type of community care, including home health care. Interaction terms were entered into the final model (widowhood * late life migration), but were not statistically significant.

TABLE 2. Descriptive Statistics for Mexican American Elderly Widows and Widowers

Variables	Widowed	
	Male %	Female %
Demographics		
Age (years)		
65-69	21.9	26.3
70-79	38.3	43.0
80 and over	39.9	30.8
Education (years)		
0	26.0	21.2
1-6	57.5	56.3
7-11	12.2	15.3
12	2.8	4.7
13 or more	1.7	2.5
Age at Migration (years)		
1-19	21.3	15.9
20-49	19.0	18.7
50 and over	12.1	11.4
Native Born	47.7	54.0
Spanish (Language of Interview)	77.1	81.0
Length of Widowhood		
Newly widowed	6.0	8.8
Living Arrangements		
Live alone	46.8	50.0
Others–head	23.4	30.2
Others–non-head	26.6	23.0
Health Care and Functioning		
Physical Disability		
Limitations on basic activities of daily living	15.1	19.5
Mental Health		
Cognitive Dysfunction		
Severe	10.6	7.0
Mild	38.8	38.8
Psychological Distress	24.6	28.3

Variables	Widowed	
	Male %	Female %
Nursing Home Use		
Ever in nursing facility	16.9	10.1**
Physician visits (mean)[1]	4.4	8.1***
Socio-Economic Situation		
A great deal of financial strain	8.7	15.3*
Poverty ratio		
Less than 1	47.0	55.4
1-1.4	38.3	34.7
1.5-2.0	7.1	4.5
More than 2.0	7.7	5.4
Insurance Coverage		
Medicaid	25.7	34.9***
Private	3.3	6.5
Medicare only	61.2	44.6
None/don't know	9.8	14.0
Assets (time-one)		
Home ownership	57.4	54.2
Private Pension	17.7	9.9**
Social Support		
Instrumental		
A lot	62.1	68.0*
Some	11.5	13.7
A little	26.4	18.3
Socioemotional		
A lot	61.3	65.8***
Some	18.7	14.9
A little	31.9	19.7
Program Participation		
Food stamps	3.3	7.5*
Any social service use	15.3	29.2***
Community-based care	8.7	15.4*
Home health care	8.7	19.7***
Unweighted N	**(183)**	**(773)**

*p ≤ .05
**p ≤ .01
***p ≤ .001
[1]t-test of significance

TABLE 3. Logistic Regressions of Home and Community-Based Long-Term Care Use by Wave Four

Variable	Any Social Service Use	Home Health Care Use	Community Care Use
Widow (vs. widower)	.84***	1.06***	.59*
Age (years)			
70-79	.19	.40	.05
80 and over	−.24	.27	−.41
Age at migration			
Late life	−.60*	−.76*	−.82*
Spanish Interview	.18	.34	.30
Health and Functioning			
Psychological distress	−.33	−.49*	−.20
Cognitive			
Mild	.12	.15	.06
Severe	.01	−.14	.01
ADL limitation	−.07	.17	.00
Social Support			
Instrumental			
A lot	.06	.16	.21
Some	−.32	−.11	−.46
Socioemotional		.07	
A lot	−.15	−.26	.46
Some	−.20	−.15	.36
Proportion in Category 1	.277	.185	.144
N	(878)	(881)	(880)

*p ≤ .05
**p ≤ .01
***p ≤ .001

Surprisingly, social support does not predict any type of community care utilization. But, ancillary analyses (not shown) indicated that having family members, especially daughters, to rely on for support reduced the probability of institutionalization. As anticipated, the analyses demonstrated that the very old, the frail, and individuals with ADL disability were more likely than non-ADL disabled persons to use a nursing facility between 1995 to 2001.

In the final analyses, we examine the influence of significant structural factors, namely, insurance status, a known barrier for inhibiting home health care service utilization. The data in Table 4 address potential differences in use by Medicaid participation. Large differences are revealed between widows and widowers in nursing facility use for welfare recipients.

The results indicate that among Medicaid recipients, widows were more likely than widowers to use senior services, community-based services, and home health care. On the other hand, widowers who had received Medicaid at time one had a greater likelihood of institutionalization than female widowed welfare recipients.

DISCUSSION

In the years to come the population over 65 will consist increasingly of minority group members, many of whom will have faced life-long economic disadvantages that increase their vulnerability in old age. Given their higher fertility and relatively favorable mortality experiences, Mexican-origin individuals are an ever-increasing segment of that growth and given the mortality advantage of women, most of those individuals will eventually be widows. In order to begin to understand the lives of older individuals, detailed longitudinal studies of specific groups, such as that employed here, will be necessary. Cross-sectional studies of large samples containing multiple groups can be useful, but the findings of such studies can be superficial. The identification of the commonalities and differences in the needs of specific groups of elderly individuals requires a detailed examination of those needs in context.

TABLE 4. Long-Term Care Utilization for Welfare Recipients in the Older Mexican American Widowed Population by Gender[1]

Type of Long-Term Care Service	Widowers	Widows	Significance	Cramer's V
Any Senior Services	18.8	38.0	p = .001	.150
Home Health Care	11.3	24.9	p = .008	.120
Community-Based Only	10.0	22.6	p = .011	.115
Nursing Facility	23.8	10.0	p = .001	−.155
N	(80)	(408)		

[1]Note: Received Supplemental Security Income and/or Medicaid benefits at baseline interview.

Our results reveal that the predictors of community care and nursing home use are similar to those found for other groups in other studies. Yet certain patterns may be unique to this group. We find that frail and disabled elderly Mexican American widows are more likely than widowers to use community care. The descriptive statistics illustrate that, by and large, in this group widows resemble widowers in terms of demographic characteristics and health profiles. However, among older Mexican Americans, widows differ substantially from widowers in the following ways: they reported fewer economic resources, more financial strain, and a greater willingness to receive welfare. All of these factors combined may increase the widow's perception that she needs support and is entitled to receive community-based long-term care services.

Our data indicate that widows are less likely than widowers to enter a nursing home. One reason suggested in the literature is the availability of family caregivers and the greater probability that women will live with their families than men. The literature suggests consistent patterns in caregiving and living arrangements in the older Hispanic population, and that a preference for or reliance on family is associated with nativity, age at migration, and gender (Angel et al., 1996). The 1982 Caregiver supplement to the National Long Term Care Survey indicates that regardless of the level of caregiving, most is performed by women (Stone, Cafferata, and Sangl, 1987). The multivariate findings on the determinants of the community-based long-term care repertoire suggest that as with other groups, increasing labor force participation by adult daughters means that they are not available to provide routine care to parents. Therefore, Latina daughters may facilitate their mother's use of community care services because of their own inability to perform much-needed caregiving tasks, including assistance with transportation and shopping (Montgomery and Datwyler, 1990).

Even among welfare recipients, widows were more likely than widowers to use community care services. Men may be less likely to use community-based services because of their lower propensity to ask for assistance from agency heads, doctors, and other health care professionals. This may be a function of a lower use of medical care, in general, among widowers. Widows, on the other hand, may find out about senior services more readily from friends, neighbors, and relatives because they have more cohesive informal networks and social ties than widowers (Antonucci, Lansford, and Schaberg, 2001).

It appears then that the Latino elderly population is more diverse than the literature portrays. Although we do not know for sure, one possible explanation is that widows tend to face fewer barriers to community care because of their greater awareness of and access to services. Lower utilization of community-based services among widowers may be a function of what Aranda and Torres (1999) refer to as a sense of "orgullo"–pride. Widowers may not be receptive to senior services. They may feel that requesting help threatens their ego, and consequently resent receiving any assistance from a case manager. These findings are intriguing, and call for further research to better understand the cultural barriers to senior services.

In conclusion, much work remains to more clearly identify the key barriers to community care for both Latina and Latino elders. Policy makers will need to consider community-based alternatives as we recognize the challenges of providing long-term care for disabled minority populations. Certainly, other factors impede the use of services, including lack of kin availability, inferior local long-term care infrastructure, and non-culturally competent service providers. Given the disproportional burden of caregiving in the Latino population, further research is called for to develop practical solutions in addressing the growing need for elder care in the Latino population.

REFERENCES

Anderton, D. L., Barrett, R. E., & Bogue, D. J. (1997). *The population of the United States*. New York: Free Press.

Angel, J. L., & Angel, R. J. (1992). Age at migration, social connections, and well-being among elderly Hispanics. *Journal of Aging and Health, 4*, 480-499.

Angel, J. L., & Angel, R. J. (1998). Mexican Americans in the southwestern United States. *Journal of Cross-Cultural Gerontology, 13*, 281-290.

Angel, J. L., Angel, R. J., & Markides, K. S. (2000). Late life immigration, changes in living arrangements and headship status among older Mexican-origin individuals. *Social Science Quarterly, 81*, 389-403.

Angel, J. L., Angel, R. J., McClelland, J., & Markides, K. S. (1996). Nativity, declining health, and preferences in living arrangement among elderly Mexican Americans: Implications for long-term care. *The Gerontologist, 13*, 281-290.

Angel, R. J., & Angel, J. L. (1996). The extent of private and public health insurance coverage among adult Hispanics. *The Gerontologist, 36*, 332-340.

Angel, R. J., & Angel, J. L. (1997). *Who will care for us? Aging and long-term care in multicultural America*. New York: New York University Press.

Angel, R. J., & Tienda, M. (1982). Determinants of extended household structure: Cultural patterns in economic need? *American Journal of Sociology, 87*, 1360-1383.

Antonucci, T. C., Lansford, J. E., & Schaberg, L. (2001). Widowhood and illness: A comparison of social network characteristics in France, Germany, Japan, and the United States. *Psychology and Aging, 16*, 655-665.

Aranda, M. P., & Torres, M. S. (1999). Self-reported barriers to the use of community-based, long-term care services. In M. Sotomayor & A. Garcia (Eds.), *La familia: Traditions and change (pp. 45-66). Washington, DC: National Hispanic Council on Aging.*

Barrett, A. E. (2000). Marital trajectories and mental health. *Journal of Health and Social Behavior, 41,* 451-464.

Carr, D., House, J. S., & Kessler, R. C. (2000). Marital quality and psychological adjustment to widowhood among older adults: A longitudinal analysis. *Journal of Gerontology, Series B: Psychological Sciences and Social Sciences 55B,* S197-S207.

Ferraro, K. F. (1984). Widowhood and social participation in later life: Isolation or compensation? *Research on Aging, 6,* 451-468.

Fields, J. & Casper, L. M. (2001). America's families and living arrangements. *Current Population Reports,* P-20 537, Table A-1. Retrieved July 5, 2002, from the U.S. Census Bureau Web site: *http://www.census.gov/population/socdemo/hh-fam/p20-537/2000/tabA1.pdf.*

Fitzpatrick, C. S., & Entmacher, J. (2000). Widows, poverty, and Social Security policy options. *Social Security Brief No. 9.* Washington, DC: National Academy of Social Insurance.

Holden, K. C., & Smock, P. J. (1991). The economic costs of marital dissolution: Why do women bear a disproportionate cost? *Annual Review of Sociology, 17,* 51-78.

Holden, K. C., & Kuo, D. (1996). Complex marital histories and economic well-being: The continuing legacy of divorce and widowhood as the HRS cohort approaches retirement. *The Gerontologist, 36,* 383-390.

Hurd, M., & Wise, D. (1989). The wealth and poverty of widows: Assets before and after the husband's death. In D. Wise (Ed.), *The economics of aging* (pp. 177-199). Chicago, IL: The University of Chicago Press.

Lee, G., & Angel, R. J. (2002). Living arrangements and Supplemental Security Income use among elderly Asians and Hispanics in the United States: The role of nativity and citizenship. *Journal of Ethnic and Migration Studies, 2,* 555-563.

Lynam, M. J. (1985). Support networks developed by immigrant women. *Social Science and Medicine, 21,* 327-333.

Montgomery, R. J. V., & Datwyler, M. M. (1990). Women and men in the caregiving role. *Generations, 14,* 34-38.

Stone, R., Cafferata, G. L., & Sangl, J. (1987). Caregivers of the frail elderly: A national profile. *The Gerontologist, 27,* 616-626.

Umberson, D., Wortman, C. B., & Kessler, R. C. (1992). Widowhood and depression: Explaining long-term gender differences in vulnerability. *Journal of Health and Social Behavior, 33,* 10-24.

U.S. Bureau of the Census. (2001). *Annual demographic survey, March CPS.* Retrieved July 25, 2002, from *http://ferret.bls.census.gov/macro/032001/pov/new01_001.htm.*

Utz, R. L., Carr, D., Nesse, R., & Wortman, C. B. (2002). The effect of widowhood on older adults' social participation: An evaluation of activity, disengagement, and continuity theories. *The Gerontologist, 42,* 522-533.

Wallace, S. P., & Lew-Ting, C. (1992). Getting by at home: Community-based long-term care of Latino elders. *Western Journal of Medicine, 157,* 337-44.

Wallace, S. P., Levy-Storms, L., & Ferguson, L. R. (1995). Access to paid in-home assistance among disabled elderly people: Do Latinos differ from non-Latino Whites? *American Journal of Public Health, 85,* 970-975.

Wallace, S. P., Campbell, K., & Lew-Ting, C. (1994). Structural barriers to the use of formal in-home services by elderly Latinos. *Journal of Gerontology: Social Sciences, 49,* S253-S263.

Wolf, D., Freedman, V., & Soldo, B. (1997). The division of family labor: Care for elderly parents. *Journal of Gerontology: Social Sciences, 52B,* 102-109.

Zick, C. D., & Smith, K. R. (1991). Patterns of economic change surrounding the death of a spouse. *Journal of Gerontology: Social Sciences, 46,* S310-S320.

Transitions to Supported Environments in England and Wales Among Elderly Widowed and Divorced Women: The Changing Balance Between Co-Residence with Family and Institutional Care

Karen Glaser, PhD
Emily Grundy, PhD
Kevin Lynch, BSc

SUMMARY. In this article we examine changes in the proportion of older widowed and divorced women in England and Wales moving from

Address correspondence to: Dr. Karen Glaser, Age Concern Institute of Gerontology, King's College London, Waterloo Bridge Wing, Franklin-Wilkins Building, Waterloo Road, London SE1 9NN (E-mail: karen.glaser@kcl.ac.uk).

The authors thank the Office for National Statistics for access to ONS Longitudinal Study data and colleagues in the former LS User Support Programme (funded by ESRC, grant reference no. H/507/255142) at the Institute of Education, University of London for their help and advice. All ONS Longitudinal Study (ONS LS) data remains Crown Copyright and the authors alone are responsible for their interpretation.

The research reported here was funded by the ESRC as part of its Population and Household Change programme, Grant Reference Number L31523018.

[Haworth co-indexing entry note]: "Transitions to Supported Environments in England and Wales Among Elderly Widowed and Divorced Women: The Changing Balance Between Co-Residence with Family and Institutional Care." Glaser, Karen, Emily Grundy, and Kevin Lynch. Co-published simultaneously in *Journal of Women & Aging* (The Haworth Press, Inc.) Vol. 15, No. 2/3, 2003, pp. 107-126; and: *Widows and Divorcees in Later Life: On Their Own Again* (ed: Carol L. Jenkins) The Haworth Press, Inc., 2003, pp. 107-126. Single or multiple copies of this article are available for a fee from The Haworth Document Delivery Service [1-800-HAWORTH, 9:00 a.m. - 5:00 p.m. (EST). E-mail address: docdelivery@haworthpress.com].

'independent' to two kinds of 'supported' household–supported private households and institutions–during the decades 1971-81 and 1981-91. Our main aim was to see whether observed increases in institutionalisation over this period were the result of a decreased propensity to move to the households of relatives. We used the ONS Longitudinal Study, a record linkage study including individual level data from the 1971, 1981 and 1991 censuses of England and Wales. A multinomial logit model was used to investigate the correlates of transitions from independent to supported private households versus institutions among elderly widowed and divorced women. While the overall rate of transitions to join either supported private households or institutions was largely the same in the two decades, the balance between the two shifted markedly in favour of transitions to institutions. In terms of the limited range of covariates it was possible to consider, owner-occupiers were significantly more likely than tenants to move to supported private households than to institutions. *[Article copies available for a fee from The Haworth Document Delivery Service: 1-800-HAWORTH. E-mail address: <docdelivery@haworthpress.com> Website: <http://www.HaworthPress.com> © 2003 by The Haworth Press, Inc. All rights reserved.]*

KEYWORDS. Divorced and widowed older women, living arrangements, ONS Longitudinal Study, England and Wales, institutions

INTRODUCTION

The well-documented increase in the proportions of older people living alone, and conversely, the marked decline in intergenerational co-residence (Börsch-Supan, 1990; Elman & Uhlenberg, 1995; Kramarow, 1995; Sundström, 1994; Waehrer & Crystal, 1995), has led to concerns that family support for elderly people is diminishing. If true, such a trend has particular implications for women, who constitute the majority of the older population. First, given gender differences in mortality which favour women, and the common pattern of women marrying older spouses, a higher proportion of women than men experience the death of a spouse. Women are also less likely than are men to remarry after widowhood or divorce (Haskey, 1999) and so far fewer older women than men of the same age have the support of a spouse. This suggests that older women may potentially rely to a greater extent on intergenerational support from children than their male peers. Additionally, an extensive literature suggests that kin relationships are more important for women than men throughout the life course reflecting the gendered nature of domestic and employment roles, and perhaps women's greater need for kin support, as well as their greater role as supporters of kin (Gerstel & Gallagher, 1993). In older age groups women's need for family support may be greater than that of men not only because of the lesser availability of a spouse, referred to above, but also because of women's higher risks of poverty, poor health and disability (Arber & Ginn, 1995; Grundy, 1998; Kinsella & Gist, 1998). In this article we examine changes in the proportion of older widowed and divorced women in England and Wales moving from 'independent' to two kinds of 'supported' household–supported private households and institutions–during the decades 1971-81 and 1981-91. Our main aim was to see whether observed increases in institutionalization over this period (Grundy & Glaser, 1997) appeared to be the result of a decreased propensity to move to the households of relatives.

Of course we recognise that many of the influences underlying the trend toward residential independence identified in the literature, such as changes in the economic ability of elderly people to maintain separate households; possible improvements in the health status of older persons; and better transport and communications systems, which may have made it easier to receive help from outside the household (Kobrin, 1976; McGarry & Schoeni, 2000; Michael, Fuchs & Scott, 1980; Pampel, 1992), are positive developments which may have enabled more elderly women to meet aspirations for 'intimacy at a distance' rather than having to live with younger relatives (Rosenmayr & Köckeis, 1963). However, numerous studies have shown that deteriorating health and widowhood are strongly associated with changes in both residence and household composition (Al-Hamad, Flowerdew & Hayes, 1997; Longino, Jackson, Zimmerman & Bradsher, 1991; Speare & McNally, 1992), and for the minority of elderly people with serious disabilities and high 'short interval' support needs, assistance provided from outside the household may be inadequate. Intra-household care provided by a spouse is not an option for widowed and divorced women. In these circumstances co-residence with other relatives or a move to institutional care may be the only alternatives. It is possible that changes during the 1980s, including increasing preferences for professional rather than family help (Daatland, 1990), and improvements in standards and amenities in nursing and residential homes, made institutional care a more acceptable alternative to family care for those with heavy support needs in Britain (Laing, Saper & Buisson, 1999).

Previous work using census micro-data from the Office for National Statistics (ONS) Longitudinal Study (LS), found that, after controlling for age, marital status and housing tenure, the risk of transition from a private household to an institution was some 33-52% higher between 1981-1991 than between 1971-1981, which we hypothesised might be associated with a decline in co-residence with family members (Grundy & Glaser, 1997). In this article we use the same data set to examine transitions from independent living arrangements (living alone or with a spouse only) to supported private households (mostly those living with adult ever-married children) or institutions among elderly women who were widowed or divorced at the end of the 1971-81 and 1981-91 decades. Specifically, we examined whether transitions among older widowed and divorced women to the two types of supported environment considered–(1) supported private households and (2) institutions–both increased in the second decade (between 1981-91) or whether increases in transitions to institutional residence were accompanied by decreases in transitions to supported private households. Socioeconomic differentials in household transitions between the two decades were also examined.

DATA AND METHODS

The ONS Longitudinal Study (LS)

The LS is based on a 1% sample of the population of England and Wales enumerated in the 1971 census. Through record linkage, the 1981 and 1991 Census records of sample members have been added to the dataset together with routinely collected data on births and deaths. The LS is a moving sample; some members are lost through emigration and death, and others are 'recruited' through the addition of 1% of immigrants and new births. Cross-sectional analyses for 1971, 1981, and 1991 refer to separate but overlapping populations of people who were present at each (or all) of the censuses, whereas longitudinal analyses between 1971-81 and 1981-91 refer to survivors: those individuals in the sample at the beginning of the interval who were still there at the end. Cross-sequential analyses are also based on separate but overlapping populations, as individuals enumerated in all three censuses will be present in the longitudinal analyses for both the 1971-81 and 1981-91 decades.

The analyses in this article focus on longitudinal data comparing transitions in living arrangements among widowed and divorced women in the 1971-81 and 1981-91 time periods. The samples for both intervals (1971-81 and 1981-91) are based on women who were widowed or divorced at the end of the reference period. Marital status at the end of the reference period was chosen in preference to initial status, or a change in marital status, as it was thought to provide a better indicator of marital status at the time of the household transition.

Definitions and Typology

Private *households* in the Census, and so in the LS, are defined as groups of co-residents who share a dwelling and have common housekeeping. The term 'private' is used to distinguish these households from 'non private' households–largely institutions. In common with most statistical offices, ONS categorises *families* in strictly nuclear terms to include married couples with or without their never-married children (of any age); lone parents with never-married children; and grandparents living with never-married grandchildren where the intervening generation is absent. In these analyses we have treated cohabiting opposite sex couples as married. *Family households* are households including at least one family; they may also include other people who are not part of the family. For example, a widow living with a divorced daughter and the daughter's never-married child would be counted as living in a lone parent household, but would not be considered a part of the lone parent family. These definitions, although widely used in censuses and surveys, are probably not congruent with popular ideas of 'family.' We use the standard definitions as building blocks for the categories we derive in order to achieve clarity and consistency.

In earlier work on transitions to supported private households using the LS (based on the data then available from the 1971 and 1981 censuses) we developed a simple typology which distinguished independent from supported households (Grundy, 1993). In the former category we included those living alone or with just a spouse and the latter category included those living with ever-married adult children, other relatives (other than a spouse or an ever-married child) or non-relatives. The terms independent and supported were, therefore, used as shorthand to refer to the availability of intra-household support from someone other than a spouse. This dichotomy, of course, represents a simplification as nearly everybody in all age groups relies to some extent on others for instrumental, emotional and financial support. Furthermore, we recognise that it cannot be assumed that elderly people living with an ever-married adult child are necessarily the recipients, rather than the providers, of support (Speare & Avery, 1993; Ward, Logan & Spitze, 1992). Nevertheless, it was felt that such a dichotomy facilitates the analysis of the determinants of transitions in living arrangements which are more likely to be associated with the support needs of the elderly person.

Improvements in the organisation of the LS datasets, and the ability to identify relationships within households, have allowed us to examine in more detail the composition of supported private households. In elaborating the typology of independent/supported private households used here, we took account of the following four criteria: the type of household; whether the elderly person was a member of the family within the household; relationship to co-residents (distinguishing children, other relatives, and non-relatives); and 'headship' of the household. The term 'household head' has not been used in the census since 1971 but a 'reference person' is identified in census analyses, this is the first adult on the census form (Hattersley & Creeser, 1995). Comparisons between the 1971 and 1981 censuses indicated that the correspondence between 'reference person' and 'household head' was close (Grundy, 1993). This typology uses the ONS definitions of household, family and family household explained above.

Institutions

Institutions are defined in the UK censuses as communal establishments where meals and services are provided (Hattersley & Creeser, 1995). The predominant types of institution in which elderly people live are residential homes for elderly people, nursing homes and (to a reducing extent) long stay hospital wards. Sheltered (warden assisted) housing for elderly people is not classed as institutional unless individual cooking facilities are available to fewer than half the residents (Hattersley & Creeser, 1995). In Britain there is much less use of nursing homes for short convalescent or rehabilitative stays than in the U.S. and we restricted our analyses to those designated as residents (rather than visitors) of an institution. General practice is to classify someone enumerated in an institution as a 'resident' if she or he has been there for at least six months and does not have an address elsewhere (Hattersley & Creeser, 1995).

Supported Private Households

Elderly people living with others in a non-family household, and those in family households but not themselves part of the family or, if part of the family, not the head or spouse of the head of household, were designated as living in supported private households. This category included, for example, elderly people living with a sibling (a non-family household); elderly widows living with a married daughter and the daughters' family (in a family household but not part of the family); and lone parents living with a never-married child where the latter was the head of household (for more detail on how the independent/supported typology was created see Glaser et al., 1997). Assignment of lone parents to the independent or supported categories was difficult, as in some cases the elderly parent may be providing rather than receiving support (Sundström, 1987). Therefore, in accordance with earlier work, it was decided that the LS member in a lone parent household would be allocated to the independent category if he/she was part of the lone parent family and the head of the household, and to the supported group if otherwise (Grundy, 1991). This interpretation is supported by analyses of the association between household relationships and migration which show that household heads were less likely to change address in the intercensal period than non-household heads, and that high proportions of the latter had moved–that is they had left their own home to move in with a relative (Al-Hamad et al., 1997; Grundy, 1993; Hayes & Al-Hamad, 1997). Again we restricted our analyses to permanent residents of households, rather than those enumerated there while paying a short-term visit.

Independent Households

In the longitudinal analyses which examined transitions between independent and supported private households among widowed or divorced women at the end of the reference period, we considered only women living in the two predominant types of independent household at the start of the interval: (1) those living alone and (2) those living only with a spouse (and no-one else), as numbers in the other independent living arrangements identified were too small for separate analysis.

Analysis Plan

The analyses in this article are based on longitudinal data comparing the 1971-81 and 1981-91 time periods. The age groups used refer to the LS member's age at the beginning of the decade; e.g., sample members who were 65-74 in 1971 would be 75-84 in 1981.

The first part of the analysis presented here is largely descriptive. We show the distribution of elderly women by marital status and household type at the end of the reference period in the two decades considered (1971-81 and 1981-91). Transition rates for 1971-81 and 1981-91, from independent households at the start of the reference period to either supported private households or institutions by the end, are shown for widowed and divorced women. In the second part of the analysis, for women who were widowed or divorced at the end of both periods, we modelled transitions to supported private households or institutions for the two time periods (1971-81 and 1981-91) for those who were in independent households at the start of the reference period. The dependent variable was household type (independent, supported private, or institutional) at the end of the 1971-81 or 1981-91 interval. Given that information was only collected at census, it is not possible to establish when within the decade any change occurred or the number of such changes. The independent variables included in the model were age group (with 65-69 being the reference category) and housing tenure (social sector and private tenants with owner-occupiers as the reference category) at the start of each interval. This co-variate was used as an indicator of socioeconomic status. In Britain, housing tenure is strongly associated with other socioeconomic indicators, such as income and occupationally derived social class, and has the advantage over the latter of being available and applicable for the whole elderly population (including, for example, very old widows with no past labour market involvement). Home ownership also provides an indicator of wealth and, as discussed later, this may have some influence on decisions about moving to institutional care. Information on income is unfortunately not collected in the UK Censuses and that available on educational status only distinguishes, in the time periods considered here, the small minority with higher level qualifications from the rest. A measure of health status, based on a question concerning limiting long-term illness, was also included in the analysis of the 1981-91 interval (as the variable was only available in the 1991 census). This question required respondents to provide a subjective assessment of their health (i.e., 'Does this person have any long-term illness, health problem or handicap which limits his/her daily activities or the work he/she can do? Include problems which are due to old age.') (Hattersley & Creeser, 1995).

A multinomial logit model was fitted in order to examine the probability distribution across the three possible categories of household at the end of the interval (0 = independent household; 1 = supported private household; 2 = institution).

RESULTS

Table 1 shows the distribution of the samples used in the analysis by marital status and age group in, respectively, 1981 and 1991. These distributions, and those in the rest of the analysis, refer to LS sample members who were, in the case of the earlier period or date, present in the LS, and at the latter date were widowed or divorced. The proportion of 75-84-year-old women who were married was slightly higher in 1991 than in 1981. This reflects both the fact that after a century or more in which women's mortality declined more than that of men, there have recently been greater improvements in male than female mortality which has delayed widowhood and offset increases in divorce (Grundy, 1998), and the small proportion of never-married women in the latter cohort. This is because marriage rates rose in the mid-decades of the twentieth century so that the proportions married are currently higher among the

TABLE 1. Percentage Distribution of Women Aged 75 and Over by Age Group and Marital Status, England and Wales, 1981 and 1991

	Age at Census					
	75-84		85+		75+	
Marital status	1981	1991	1981	1991	1981	1991
Single	13	9	14	13	13	10
Married	25	28	8	9	22	24
Widowed/Divorced	62	62	77	78	65	66
Base = 100%	14,029	16,128	3,376	5,031	17,405	21,159

Source: Authors' own analysis of ONS LS

young elderly population than among the oldest old (Grundy, 1999; Haskey, 1993; ONS, 1999).

TYPE OF INDEPENDENT/SUPPORTED PRIVATE HOUSEHOLD AT THE END OF THE INTERVAL

Table 2 shows the distribution of elderly widowed and divorced women by household type (independent or supported) in 1981 and 1991. The proportion of the elderly widowed and divorced population in independent households was higher in 1991 than ten years earlier, largely reflecting the widely reported rise in solitary living among older people (Börsch-Supan, 1990; Elman & Uhlenberg, 1995; Kramarow, 1995; Sundström, 1994; Waehrer & Crystal, 1995). Thus among divorced and

TABLE 2. Percentage Distribution of Widowed and Divorced Women by Age Group and Household Type, England and Wales, 1981 and 1991

	Age at Census					
	75-84		85+		75+	
Household type	1981	1991	1981	1991	1981	1991
Independent						
Solitary	68	74	47	56	63	69
[a]Head in a lone parent family	8	7	8	5	8	6
Sub-total	*76*	*81*	*55*	*61*	*71*	*75*
Supported						
Not head in lone parent family	2	2	3	2	2	2
Lives with ever-married child	11	7	20	10	13	8
Lives with other relative	3	2	3	2	3	2
Lives with non-relative	2	1	2	1	2	1
Sub-total	*18*	*12*	*28*	*15*	*20*	*13*
[b]Other	6	7	17	24	8	12
Base = 100%	8,732	10,031	2,614	3,917	11,346	13,948

Note: [a]This category includes the few women cohabitors in family households.
[b]The other category includes mostly those individuals living in institutions, but also includes a few servants in 1981, and small numbers of elderly people living with their parents.
Source: Authors' own analysis of ONS LS

widowed women aged 85 and over the proportion in independent households increased from 55% in 1981 to 61% in 1991. Conversely, the proportions of widowed and divorced women in this age group in supported private households declined markedly from 28% in 1981 compared with 15% in 1991. Within this category the largest decrease occurred in the proportions living with an ever-married child, declining from 20% in 1981 to 10% by 1991.

TRANSITIONS TO SUPPORTED PRIVATE HOUSEHOLDS AND INSTITUTIONS

Analyses of transitions between 1971-81 are obviously restricted to those still alive and in the sample in 1981; similarly, analyses of second decade transitions are restricted to those still in the sample in 1991 (including sample members added between 1971 and 1981). As attrition rates through death are high in these age groups, these survivors represent a selected group (Grundy, 1987). Moreover, as we do not have information on the timing or frequency of intercensal household transitions even for survivors, the transition rates presented are underestimates of the true extent of transition over the relevant decade as in the case of a woman who, for example, moved to live with a daughter and then to a nursing home in one decade; information on the first transition is not available.

In the following analyses we examine differences between the two decades in transitions from independent households to supported private households or to institutions among women who were widowed or divorced at the end of the reference period. As our aim was to examine transitions from independent to supported settings (either with relatives or in institutions) only those who were living alone or with a spouse only at the beginning of the decade were considered (numbers in the other types of independent household considered were too small for separate analyses).

Table 3 shows the percentage of widowed and divorced women in supported private households and institutions at the end of the decade by age and type of independent household at the beginning of the decade for the 1971-81 and 1981-91 periods. Overall, as would be expected, the proportions of widowed and divorced women who by the end of either the 1971-81 or 1981-91 interval were in supported private households and in institutions increased with age.

TABLE 3. Transitions to Supported Private Households (SPH) and Institutions Among Widowed and Divorced Women at the End of the Interval, by Age and Type of Independent Household at the Start of the Interval, 1971-81 and 1981-91, England and Wales

Age and type of independent household at the start of the interval		Percentage in supported private households or institutions at the end of the interval							
		SPH		Institution		SPH or Institution		Ratio SPH/Institutions	
		71-81	81-91	71-81	81-91	71-81	81-91	71-81	81-91
65-74	Solitary	7	5	7	8	14	13	1.0	0.6
	MC only	11	6	5	8	16	14	2.2	0.8
	Total	9	6	6	8	15	14	1.5	0.8
75+	Solitary	12	7	20	26	32	33	0.6	0.3
	MC only	19	9	21	24	40	33	0.9	0.4
	Total	14	7	20	26	34	33	0.7	0.3
65+	Solitary	9	6	10	14	19	20	0.9	0.4
	MC only	12	7	8	11	20	18	1.5	0.6
	Total	10	6	9	13	19	19	1.1	0.5

Note: MC only = married couple only; SPH = supported private households. N = 7,858 for widowed and divorced women in the 1971-81 interval; N = 10,928 for widowed and divorced women in the 1981-91 interval.
Source: Authors' own analysis of ONS LS

The proportion of elderly widowed and divorced women who were living alone at the beginning of the interval, and who were resident in supported private households at the end, decreased between the 1971-81 and 1981-91 time periods. For example, among widowed and divorced women at the end of the interval, who were aged 75 and over at the start, 12% of those who were in solitary households in 1971 were in supported private households by 1981; by comparison, 7% of women in this category living alone in 1981 were in supported private households by 1991 (Table 3).

Overall, although similar proportions of widowed and divorced women between the two decades entered either supported private households or institutions, what changed dramatically between the two time periods was the balance between these two household types. For example, among women who were widowed or divorced at the end of the relevant interval, and aged 75 and over and living alone at its start, about 32% in both decades were in either a supported private household or an institution by the end of the interval (Table 3). However, the ratio of moves to supported private households to moves to institutions halved over the two decades from 0.6:1 to 0.3:1.

MULTIVARIATE ANALYSIS

The descriptive analyses presented above demonstrate the importance of age as an influence on transitions in living arrangements. In addition, previous work has shown that social housing tenants had lower rates of transition to supported private households than owner-occupiers or private sector tenants, suggesting a positive association between resources and moving in with relatives (Grundy, 1993). Finally, as discussed above, numerous studies have found health to be an important factor affecting changes in household composition in later life.

A multinomial logit model was fitted to the data in order to enable the examination of the relative importance of each of these factors as well as their effect on one type of household versus another. The odds ratios, their confidence intervals, and level of significance are presented in Tables 4 and 5. In interpreting the odds ratios, recall that they represent the log-odds of one outcome versus another given a one-unit change in the independent variable. The outcomes considered here are the following: (1) living in an institution at the end of the interval versus living independently; (2) living in a supported private household at the end of the interval versus living independently; and (3) living in a supported private household at the end of the interval versus living in an institution. Only widowed and divorced women at the end of the interval, who were aged 65 or over at the start and were then either living alone or just with their spouse, were included in the analysis.

The second and third columns of Table 4 show the odds ratios of entering an institution versus remaining in an independent household for the 1971-81 and 1981-91 decades among widowed and divorced women at the end of the interval who were in independent households at the beginning of the decade. Age had a significantly positive effect on entry into an institution versus remaining in an independent household in the two time periods, i.e., the older the woman's age, the greater the odds that she would enter an institution rather than be still living independently at the end of the interval. In the 1981-91 decade, tenants in social sector housing were more likely than owner-occupiers to be in institu-

TABLE 4. Multinomial Regression Model of Household Transitions Among Widowed and Divorced Women at the End of the Interval, 1971-81 and 1981-91, England and Wales

		Transitions					
		Institution vs. Independent		Supported vs. Independent		Supported vs. Institution	
At start of interval		71-81	81-91	71-81	81-91	71-81	81-91
Age							
	70-74	2.04**	2.78**	1.28**	1.17	0.63**	0.42**
		(1.65-2.51)	(2.33-3.33)	(1.07-1.53)	(0.97-1.42)	(0.48-0.82)	(0.33-0.54)
	75+	5.89**	7.55**	2.32**	1.82**	0.39**	0.24**
		(4.81-7.19)	(6.40-8.92)	(1.93-2.79)	(1.51-2.21)	(0.31-0.51)	(0.19-0.31)
Housing tenure							
Social housing tenant		1.12	1.17*	0.62**	0.74**	0.55**	0.63**
		(0.93-1.35)	(1.03-1.33)	(0.51-0.75)	(0.62-0.89)	(0.43-0.71)	(0.51-0.78)
Private renter		1.17	1.44**	0.92	0.87	0.79	0.61**
		(0.95-1.43)	(1.22-1.69)	(0.77-1.11)	(0.69-1.09)	(0.61-1.02)	(0.46-0.79)

Note: Confidence intervals are in parentheses. Reference categories are as follows: age, 65-69; tenure, owner-occupier. N = 7,849 for the 1971-81 interval; N = 10,928 for the 1981-91 interval.
*p < .05; **p < .01.
Source: Authors' own analysis of ONS LS

tions at the end of the interval than to remain in independent households. Private renters at the beginning of the second decade were also significantly more likely to enter an institution by the end of the decade than owner-occupiers.

The fourth and fifth columns look at transitions to supported private households versus remaining in independent households for those individuals aged 65 and over living independently at the start of the interval, once again by their characteristics at baseline. With respect to age, the older a woman was at the start of the interval the more likely she was to enter a supported private household rather than remain in an independent household at the end of the interval. Social housing tenants were significantly less likely to enter supported private households than to remain living independently when compared with owner-occupiers and this relationship held for both decades.

The sixth and seventh columns show the correlates of transitions to supported private households versus institutions at the end of both decades for widowed and divorced women living in independent households at the start. With regards to age, the older the age of a woman at the start of the decade the less likely she was to enter a supported private household rather than an institution by the end of the decade. Widowed and divorced women who were social housing tenants at the start of the interval were less likely than owner-occupiers to enter a supported private household versus an institution by the end of the decade for both periods. In the 1981-91 decade widowed or divorced women who were private renters were also less likely to enter supported private households rather than an institution by the end of the interval.

The addition of a census question in 1991 on limiting long-term illness enabled an examination of the effect of health on transitions to supported private households and institutions. As no information on health was included in earlier censuses, the analysis that follows is restricted to longitudinal data from the 1981-91 interval.

Table 5 repeats the multinomial model shown for the 1981-91 decade with the addition of the limiting long-term illness variable in 1991. Given the strong association between poor health and institutionalisation among the very old population (Dolinsky & Rosenwaike, 1988), it was expected that individuals in poor health would be significantly more likely to enter institutions than remain living independently, would be significantly more likely to enter supported private households than remain living independently, and would be significantly less likely to enter supported private households than institutions. This was the case as is shown in Table 5. Controlling for health status in this way showed once

TABLE 5. Multinomial Regression Model of Household Transitions Among Widowed and Divorced Women at the End of the Interval, 1981-91, England and Wales

At start of interval		Transitions 1981-91		
		Institution vs. Independent	Supported vs. Independent	Supported vs. Institution
Age				
	70-74	2.38**	1.13	0.48**
		(1.98-2.85)	(0.93-1.38)	(0.37-0.62)
	75+	5.37**	1.69**	0.32**
		(4.52-6.38)	(1.39-2.06)	(0.25-0.40)
Housing tenure				
Social sector tenant		0.98	0.71**	0.72**
		(0.85-1.12)	(0.59-0.85)	(0.58-0.90)
Private renter		1.37**	0.86	0.62**
		(1.16-1.63)	(0.68-1.08)	(0.48-0.82)
Health				
Limiting long-term illness		19.7**	1.48**	0.08**
		(15.01-25.89)	(1.26-1.74)	(0.05-0.10)

Note: Confidence intervals are in parentheses. Reference categories are as follows: age, 65-69; tenure, owner-occupier; limiting long-term illness, no.
N = 10,928.
*p < .05; **p < .01.
Source: Authors' own analysis of ONS LS

again the important link between health and changes in living arrangements among older people.

DISCUSSION

The results presented here show large decreases over time in the proportions of older widowed and divorced women living in what we have termed supported private households and corresponding increases in the proportions living alone. This is consistent with the well-documented trend towards greater residential independence in older age groups. We have additionally shown that transitions to supported private households were lower in 1981-91 than in the previous decade while transitions to institutions increased. As a result the overall rate of transitions to join either type of supported environment–supported private or an institution–was much the same, but the balance between the two shifted markedly. Such a finding would have been missed if our analysis had been confined to cross-sectional data on the private household population only. The advantage of the LS is both its longitudinal element and the fact that the institutionalised population is included. However, it must be acknowledged that the data set has certain weaknesses as well, notably the lack of information on other relevant factors (such as more information on health limitations) and the inability to precisely time transitions between two census points.

Several factors may underlie the apparent shift from co-residence with family members to institutional care. First, it is possible that the willingness of, for example, married daughters to accommodate frail elderly parents may have decreased and/or that elderly people have become even more reluctant to become a 'burden' to younger relatives. An important factor influencing the relative desirability (or undesirability) of institutional care as compared with co-residence with family members may also be the steady improvement in standards and amenities in nursing and residential homes (Laing et al., 1999). Importantly, too, access to institutional care in England and Wales was effectively increased during the 1980s as a result of changes in the administration of social security benefits which led to payments being made available to cover the cost of fees in residential homes (Laing, 1993). In terms of the limited range of covariates we were able to consider, it seems that owner-occupiers were more likely than tenants to move to supported private households rather than to institutions. This suggests that in England and Wales, assuming that the children of the more advantaged are themselves more likely to be advantaged, greater family socioeconomic resources may facilitate the provision of family support to an elderly relative. Policies which require elderly people with incomes over a certain level (including income from the imputed value of assets) to make a contribution to the costs of certain types of institutional care, or render them ineligible for social security payments which partially covered care costs, may also have served to make entry to an institution a less desired option for those with assets (Laing, 1993). In addition, relatives in some of these cases may prefer to provide care themselves rather than see their potential inheritance spent on nursing home fees. While the positive association between indicators of greater socioeconomic resources and intergenerational co-residence (including transitions by elderly people to supported private households) has also been found for Canada (Béland & Santé, 1987), research from the U.S. shows the reverse relationship (Hoyert, 1991; Soldo, Wolf & Agree, 1990; Wolf & Soldo, 1988). This may reflect differences in the availability of publicly provided domiciliary services, and in the financing of institutional care. In Britain, as in Sweden and the Netherlands, official policy is to avoid institutionalisation wherever possible. The National Health Service (NHS) and Community Care Act implemented in Britain in 1993 was designed to reverse perverse incentives to enter institutions. Some decline in admission rates since then has been reported (Laing et al., 1999); however, it is not yet known how this may have affected differentials in entry to an institution or moves to live with relatives. If the shift in transitions to these two types of setting observed in the data analysed here continues, then the implication is of increasing demand for institutional long-term care in England and Wales, which already has a high rate of institutionalisation within Europe (Jacobzone, 1999). The important outstanding question is what is the implication of this apparent shift for the well-being of elderly widows and divorcees? This question requires detailed information, both quantitative and qualitative, not available in the ONS LS and must be addressed in other studies.

REFERENCES

Al-Hamad, A., Flowerdew, R., & Hayes, L. (1997). Migration of Elderly People to Join Existing Households: Some Evidence from the 1991 Household Sample of Anonymised Records. *Environment and Planning A, 29*, 1243-1255.

Arber, S., & Ginn, J. (1995). *Connecting Gender and Ageing. A Sociological Approach.* Buckingham: Open University Press.

Béland, F., & Groupe de Recherche Interdisciplinaire en Santé (1987). Multigenerational Households in a Contemporary Perspective. *International Journal of Aging and Human Development, 25*, 147-166.

Börsch-Supan, A. H. (1990). A Dynamic Analysis of Household Dissolution and Living Arrangement Transitions by Elderly Americans. In D.A. Wise (Ed.), *Issues in the Economics of Aging* (pp. 89-114). Chicago: National Bureau of Economic Research.

Daatland, S. O. (1990). What Are Families For? On Family Solidarity and Preference for Help. *Ageing and Society, 10*, 1-15.

Dolinsky, A. L., & Rosenwaike, I. (1988). The Role of Demographic Factors in the Institutionalization of the Elderly. *Research on Aging, 10*(2), 235-257.

Elman, C., & Uhlenberg, P. (1995). Co-Residence in the Early Twentieth Century: Elderly Women in the United States and Their Children. *Population Studies, 49*, 501-517.

Gerstel, N., & Gallagher, S. K. (1993). Kinkeeping and Distress: Gender, Recipients of Care, and Work-Family Conflict. *Journal of Marriage and the Family, 55*, 598-607.

Glaser, K., Grundy, E., & Lynch, K. (1997). Household Transitions: Coding Independent and Supported Households among Older Persons. *UPDATE-News from the LS User Group*(18), 5-7.

Grundy, E. (1987). Household Change and Migration among the Elderly in England and Wales. *Espace, Populations, Societes, 1*, 109-123.

Grundy, E. (1991). Ageing: Age Related Change in Later Life. In M. J. Murphy, & J. Hobcraft (Eds.), *Population Research in Britain* Supplement to Population Studies (pp. 133-156).

Grundy, E. (1993). Moves into Supported Private Households among Elderly People in England and Wales. *Environment and Planning A, 25*, 1467-1479.

Grundy, E. (1998). The Epidemiology of Aging. In R. Tallis, H. Fillit, & J. C. Brocklehurst (Eds.), *Brocklehurst's Textbook of Geriatric Medicine and Gerontology* (pp. 1-17). London: Churchill Livingstone.

Grundy, E. (1999). Intergenerational Perspectives on Family and Household Change in Mid- and Later Life in England and Wales." In S. McRae (Ed.), *Changing Britain. Families and Households in the 1990s* (pp. 201-228). Oxford: Oxford University Press.

Grundy, E., & Glaser, K. (1997). Trends in, and Transitions to, Institutional Residence among Older People in England and Wales, 1971-91. *Journal of Epidemiology and Community Health, 51*, 531-540.

Haskey, J. (1993). First Marriage, Divorce, and Remarriage: Birth Cohort Analyses. *Population Trends, 72*, 24-33.

Haskey, J. (1999). Divorce and Remarriage in England and Wales. *Population Trends, 95*, 18-22.

Hattersley, L., & Creeser, R. (1995). *Longitudinal Study 1971-1991: History, Organisation and Quality of Data, Series Ls No. 7*. London: HMSO.

Hayes, L., & Al-Hamad, A. (1997). Residential Movement into Elderly Person Households: Evidence from the 1991 Household Sample of Anonymised Records. *Environment and Planning A, 29*, 1433-1447.

Hoyert, D. L. (1991). Financial and Household Exchanges between Generations. *Research on Aging, 13*(2), 205-225.

Jacobzone, S. (1999). Ageing and Care for Frail Elderly Persons: An Overview of International Perspectives. Occasional Papers no. 38. Paris: OECD.

Kinsella, K., & Gist, Y. J. (1998). Gender and Aging. Mortality and Health. International Brief 98-2. Washington, D.C.: U.S. Bureau of the Census.

Kobrin, F. E. (1976). The Primary Individual and the Family: Changes in Living Arrangements in the United States since 1940. *Journal of Marriage and the Family, 38*, 233-239.

Kramarow, E. A. (1995). The Elderly Who Live Alone in the United States: Historical Perspectives on Household Change. *Demography, 32*(3), 335-352.

Laing, W. (1993). *Financing Long-Term Care: The Crucial Debate*. London: Age Concern England.

Laing, W., Saper, P., & Laing, & Buisson. (1999). Chapter 6: Promoting the Development of a Flourishing Independent Sector Alongside Good Quality Public Services. In M. Henwood & G. Wistow (Eds.), *Evaluating the Impact of Caring for People. A Report by the Royal Commission on Long Term Care* (pp. 87-102). London: The Stationery Office.

Longino, C. F., Jackson, D. J., Zimmerman, R. S., & Bradsher, J. E. (1991). The Second Move: Health and Geographic Mobility. *Journal of Gerontology: Social Sciences, 46*(4), S218-S24.

McGarry, K., & Schoeni, R. (2000). Social Security, Economic Growth, and the Rise in the Elderly Widow's Independence in the Twentieth Century. *Demography,* *37*(2), 221-236.

Michael, R., Fuchs, V., & Scott, S. (1980). Changes in the Propensity to Live Alone. *Demography, 19*, 39-53.

Office for National Statistics (ONS). (1999). *Marriage, Divorce and Adoption Statistics. Series Fm2 No. 24.* London: The Stationery Office.

Pampel, F. C. (1992). Trends in Living Alone among the Elderly in Europe. In A. Rogers (Ed.), *Elderly Migration and Population Redistribution: A Comparative Study* (pp. 97-117). London: Belhaven Press.

Rosenmayr, L., & Köckeis, E. (1963). Propositions for a Sociological Theory of Aging and the Family. *International Social Science Journal, 15*(3), 410-426.

Soldo, B. J., Wolf, D. A., & Agree, E. M. (1990). Family, Households, and Care Arrangements of Frail Older Women: A Structural Analysis. *Journal of Gerontology: Social Sciences, 45*(6), S238-S249.

Speare, A., & Avery, R. (1993). Who Helps Whom in Older Parent-Child Families. *Journal of Gerontology: Social Sciences, 48*(2), S64-S73.

Speare, A., & McNally, J. (1992). The Relation of Migration and Household Change among Elderly Persons. In A. Rogers (Ed.), *Elderly Migration and Population Redistribution: A Comparative Study* (pp. 61-76). London: Belhaven Press.

Sundström, G. (1987). A Haven in a Heartless World? Living with Parents in Sweden and the United States, 1880-1982. *Continuity and Change, 2*, 145-187.

Sundström, G. (1994). Care by Families: An Overview of Trends. In OECD (Ed.), *Caring for Frail Elderly People. New Directions in Care* (pp. 15-55). Paris: OECD Social Policy Studies.

Waehrer, K., & Crystal, S. (1995). The Impact of Coresidence on Economic Well-Being of Elderly Widows. *Journal of Gerontology: Social Sciences, 50B*(4), S250-S258.

Ward, R., Logan, J., & Spitze, G. (1992). The Influence of Parent and Child Needs on Coresidence in Middle and Later Life. *Journal of Marriage and the Family, 54*, 209-221.

Wolf, D. A., & Soldo, B. J. (1988). Household Composition Choices of Older Unmarried Women. *Demography, 25*(3), 387-403.

Care Arrangement Choices
for Older Widows:
Decision Participants' Perspectives

Carol L. Jenkins, MPA, PhD

SUMMARY. This research examines how a wide range of care arrangement decisions for frail older women are made. Interviews were conducted with 11 older women (ten of whom are widows), nine of their family members, and six professional service providers. Maintaining the older woman's independence was identified as a major theme. While all decision participants identified it as an explicit or implicit decision-making goal, their meanings of independence were different. The older women's meanings were flexible, changing in response to changes in their physical condition and need for assistance. Adult children tended to identify their mothers as independent when they did not actually need assistance, or when they received help from other sources (e.g., home health care). Professional service providers were inclined to define independence narrowly, as avoiding nursing home placement. Minor themes

The author thanks Sarah Laditka and three anonymous reviewers for thoughtful comments on earlier drafts of this paper.

Address correspondence to: Carol L. Jenkins, East Carolina University, School of Social Work/Center on Aging, 203 Ragsdale Building, Greenville, NC 27858-4353 (E-mail: jenkinsca@mail.ecu.edu).

This research was supported in part by a Roscoe Martin Research Grant from the Maxwell School, Syracuse University.

[Haworth co-indexing entry note]: "Care Arrangement Choices for Older Widows: Decision Participants' Perspectives." Jenkins, Carol L. Co-published simultaneously in *Journal of Women & Aging* (The Haworth Press, Inc.) Vol. 15, No. 2/3, 2003, pp. 127-143; and: *Widows and Divorcees in Later Life: On Their Own Again* (ed: Carol L. Jenkins) The Haworth Press, Inc., 2003, pp. 127-143. Single or multiple copies of this article are available for a fee from The Haworth Document Delivery Service [1-800-HAWORTH, 9:00 a.m. - 5:00 p.m. (EST). E-mail address: docdelivery@haworthpress.com].

associated with independence include responsibility, reciprocity, and the family's importance in maintaining independence. These themes help to clarify the complex dynamics that take place during care arrangement decisions and explain how care arrangement choices are made. *[Article copies available for a fee from The Haworth Document Delivery Service: 1-800-HAWORTH. E-mail address: <docdelivery@haworthpress.com> Website: <http://www.HaworthPress.com>* © *2003 by The Haworth Press, Inc. All rights reserved.]*

KEYWORDS. Care arrangement decisions, independence, older widows, informal care, formal care, nursing home care

The aging of the U.S. population has interest for researchers, service providers, and policymakers. As people grow older, particularly at ages over 85, they are more likely to experience health problems and declines in physical function. Such declines make it difficult to perform normal activities of daily living (ADLs) such as bathing or dressing, and instrumental activities of daily living (IADLs), such as doing laundry or grocery shopping. While many older individuals continue to care for themselves in spite of difficulty, others need assistance. This need is met by the informal care system (e.g., spouses, children, friends), by the formal service provision system (e.g., nursing homes, home health care), or by some combination of the two. Instituting a care arrangement often involves a complex decision-making process as participants can include the older person, various family members, and often a professional service provider.

BACKGROUND

Research regarding the outcomes of care arrangement decision making is abundant (e.g., Falcone & Broyles, 1994; Logan & Spitze, 1994; Miller, McFall, & Campbell, 1994; Miner, 1995; Salive, Collins, Foley, & George, 1993). Most studies are quantitative, are modeled within a rational decision-making framework, and are focused on identifying a range of demographic, socioeconomic, and health-related factors associated with various care arrangements.

Studies investigating the process underlying care decisions often employ qualitative methods. Research on informal care decision making has explored family members' participation in the care decision and attitudes about providing care. Spouses and children have a fundamental interest in participating in the decision process, since they are responsible for much of the assistance a frail older person receives. Many adult children, particularly daughters, have strong affective ties to parents that motivate them to provide assistance to frail parents (Horowitz & Shindelman, 1983). Other children provide assistance to a parent out of a sense of duty; this is particularly so when dysfunctional relationships between children and parents have resulted in a lack of filial affection (Whitbeck, Hoyt, & Huck, 1994). Children sometimes make decisions related to caregiving without including the parent in the process. For example, Matthews and Rosner (1988) found that adult children often determined among themselves how responsibility for parent care would be divided.

Research shows that older people want to participate in decisions relating to their care, even when they are not able to obtain the care arrangement they prefer (Wetle, Levkoff, Cwikel, & Rosen, 1988). Active participation in the process leaves them more satisfied with both the decision process and with the outcome (Coulton et al., 1989). At the same time, they prefer that family members, especially spouses and children, participate in the process as well. The inclusion of family members gives older people a sense of support, and strengthens their feelings of control over the decision (Prohaska & Glasser, 1996).

The need for formal care necessarily introduces a representative of the service provision system into the decision-making process. These individuals, including social workers, physicians, and nurses, have well-established professional norms meant to guide their decision making. Relevant professional norms include protecting clients's best interests, safeguarding their autonomy, and ensuring their safety (Hennessy, 1989; High, 1988; Wetle, 1995). These issues take on added importance when surrogate decision-making is necessary, as is often the case when an older person's cognitive function has deteriorated (High & Rowles, 1995).

Existing studies of care arrangement decision making provide a foundation for understanding the decision process, but they share some limitations. First, their results are based on the perspective of one, or at most two, of the decision participants. Reliance on only some participants' perspectives of what occurs during the decision process results in an incomplete picture of care arrangement decision making. It can also result in missing the often different perceptions of the process on the part of participants (Pratt, Jones, Shin, & Walker, 1989). Second, previous studies have focused on decisions related to a specific type of care arrangement (e.g., Gonyea, 1987; Matthews & Rosner, 1988). This limits our ability to identify themes that may be common across decisions related to different types of care arrangements. This article presents results of an exploratory study examining the care arrangement decision process from the perspective of all decision participants. Themes are identified that should be explored in future research.

METHODS

Sample Selection

The choice of sample selection criteria for this study was guided by a focus on exploring complex decision-making processes and on the need to include a variety of care arrangements. Community-dwelling married people needing care are very likely to receive the bulk of their assistance from a spouse (Jenkins, 2002), which tends to simplify the care arrangement decision. Thus, only individuals who were without a spouse were included, and particular emphasis was put on recruiting participants with children as they would be likely to face a more complex decision process.

Due to the exploratory nature of the study, a small convenience sample representing people associated with five different care arrangements was chosen. Care arrangements included self-only care (i.e., self-care as the sole strategy), nursing home care, and three types of helper networks: only informal helpers, only formal helpers, and a mix of informal and formal helpers. Selection of individuals for each of these care categories differed. Individuals receiving any assistance from the formal service sector were recruited through service providers. Contact was made with the office for aging in two counties of North Carolina, with a request for assistance in identifying older persons receiving home care who met the study's eligibility criteria. Case managers in each office identified appropriate individuals and agreed to provide interviews on their perspective of the decision process. The names of family members participating in the care arrangement decisions were provided by either the older person or the case manager. Five women were recruited in this manner.

Sample members receiving nursing home care were recruited at a nursing home in one of the counties. Potential sample members identified by an intake case manager in the nursing home were screened to identify persons cognitively able and willing to participate in the study. Two women were chosen by this means for inclusion in the study. One of the women identified a son to contact for the family interview; the other had no children and no living siblings, so no family interview was held. The intake manager at the nursing home participated in the provider interview for both women.

Individuals who received assistance from only informal helpers or who received no assistance from others were identified through the author's personal acquaintances and professional contacts in the same counties. Four women were recruited for the study in this way. Each woman provided the name of a family member who had participated in the decision process and who was willing to be interviewed.

Data Collection

In-depth, semi-structured interviews were held with each study participant separately. They were conducted in person, except for five telephone interviews with adult children who lived out-of-state. Structured questionnaires were used first to gather demographic, socioeconomic, and family structure data from each older person and family member. Questions about physical and cognitive function were included in the older person's survey. Providers were asked about education and standard decision criteria.

Open-ended questions were included in each interview intended to gather detailed, qualitative data about the circumstances surrounding the need for care, the decision-making process, decision criteria, feelings about giving and receiving assistance, and satisfaction with the decision-making process and the care arrangement chosen. Conversation taking place when participants were answering open-ended questions was taped. Following each interview, field notes were made of conversation that was not taped, such as clarifying information provided while answering the survey questionnaire and after the recorder was turned off.

The Sample

The final sample consisted of 26 individuals: 11 women, nine of their family members, five case managers, and one nursing home administrator. Demographic, disability status, and care arrangement information about each woman is provided in Table 1. The women ranged in age from 65 to 88, with a mean age of 80. All but one of the women were widows with children; the other woman had never been married and had no children. There was a wide range of disability states as measured by the number of ADLs and IADLs with which the women received help.

The two women who were able to take care of themselves were the least disabled, while those women who received help from a mix of informal and formal helpers tended to be the most disabled.

Providing detailed information about each sample participant's circumstances is beyond the scope of this article. A brief description of contextual factors for several of the participants is provided in Exhibit 1,

TABLE 1. Demographic Data, Disability Status, and Care Arrangements for the Study Sample

	Age	Marital status	Number of children	Number of ADLs[a]	Number of IADLs[b]	Care arrangement
Mrs. R.	81	widow	2 sons 6 daughters	1	1	self only
Mrs. M.	76	widow	2 sons	1	1	self only
Mrs. W.	82	widow	1 son 6 stepchildren	5	na[c]	nursing home
Ms. J.	88	never married	none	3	na[c]	nursing home
Mrs. C.	85	widow	1 daughter	3	3	informal only
Mrs. B.	86	widow	2 sons	4	4	informal only
Mrs. H.	77	widow	3 daughters	6	7	mix of helpers
Mrs. P.	72	widow	2 sons	5	4	mix of helpers
Mrs. S.	84	widow	1 son 2 daughters	3	3	mix of helpers
Mrs. F.	65	widow	3 sons	4	7	mix of helpers
Mrs. L.	78	widow	1 son 1 daughter	1	4	formal only

[a]This is the number of activities of daily living for which a woman needed help. Activities include eating, dressing, bathing, getting around inside the house, using the toilet, and transferring in and out of bed.

[b]This is the number of instrumental activities of daily living for which a woman needed help. Activities include housework, laundry, preparing meals, shopping for groceries, managing money, taking medicine, and using the telephone.

[c] Data concerning IADLs was not gathered from the two participants who resided in a nursing home. Since most of the activities are performed by staff, nursing home residents would always report disability for these items.

however. The cases described were selected to be representative of the general problems facing all of the older women in the sample and of the issues discussed by study participants.

Data Analysis

The field notes and taped interviews were compiled into a written database containing detailed information about each older woman, her care arrangement, and the decision-making process. Some methodologists argue against the necessity of making literal transcriptions of taped interviews, suggesting that careful listening to interview conversations may enhance the researcher's ability to understand and analyze what respondents have to say (e.g., Bogden & Taylor, 1975; DeVault, 1999). Consequently, the taped interview conversations were listened to repeatedly, with meticulous notes taken throughout the process. Once the written database had been created, a thematic analysis was conducted (Luborsky, 1994). Content analysis and coding techniques were employed to construct a chart showing major themes, comparisons, and contrasts in the information

RESULTS

Several important themes emerged as participants discussed the factors that influenced their input into the decision-making process and the care arrangement they preferred. Underlying most of the issues discussed was the importance of maintaining the independence of the older woman, although participants attributed different meanings to independence. In related themes, participants discussed concerns about safety, responsibility for helping, the reciprocal nature of care, and the family's importance in maintaining independence.

Maintaining the Older Woman's Independence

All the participants made either implicit or explicit reference to preserving the older women's independence as one of the primary values underlying their decision making. They discussed independence in a relative, rather than absolute, sense, although they tended to use different reference points for making relative comparisons.

The older women's meanings of independence were fluid, shifting in conjunction with changes in their health status that directly affected

EXHIBIT 1. Contextual Factors for Selected Sample Participants

Mrs. W: Mrs. W., a nursing home resident for two years, has difficulty dressing, bathing, getting in and out of bed, and toileting. She gets around by propelling herself in a wheelchair. At 82, Mrs. W. has been widowed twice. She has one natural son, Frank, who lives a few hundred miles away, and visits her several times a year. Three of her six stepchildren live nearby and visit her occasionally. Before entering the nursing home, Mrs. W. lived alone in a relatively rural area. She fell on several occasions, experiencing only mild bruises. Eventually she fractured her hip in a serious fall and was hospitalized. Care plans were discussed with her son, her physician, and a social worker employed by the hospital. Frank wanted her to move in with his family, but Mrs. W refused. She said she "just couldn't think about going away forever." She could not afford to hire full-time help at home and was worried about living alone if she should fall again, so she entered a nursing home.

Mrs. C: Mrs. C., an 85-year-old widow, lives alone in one unit of a subsidized apartment complex for older individuals. She cares for herself by using equipment such as a cane, tub bars, and a raised toilet seat. Her daughter helps her manage her money, takes her on errands, and occasionally assists with housework. A year and a half prior to her interview, Mrs. C. had a hip replacement. Discharge plans were discussed among Mrs. C., her daughter, her physician, and the hospital discharge planner. In spite of concerns about her safety, Mrs. C. insisted she try returning home. She actually spent one night there with her daughter's company, but realized that she would no longer feel safe alone. Although she had learned to walk quite well again, she was worried about falling and hurting herself. In addition, she could no longer drive so she knew that she would essentially be housebound. Her daughter suggested that she move in with her family, but Mrs. C. did not want to "be on top of them all the time." She chose instead to move to the senior housing complex, which is located about 10 miles from her daughter's home.

Mrs. H: Mrs. H. is a 77-year-old widow who lives alone in her home of over 40 years. A year before her interview, she had a double knee replacement. Before she was fully recovered, she fell and broke her shoulder. These two acute health care episodes, occurring so closely together, left her experiencing difficulty with all ADLs and IADLs. She gets assistance from a mix of formal and informal helpers, including two home health aides, a physical therapist, a friend, and her three daughters. Following her shoulder injury, Mrs. H. received intensive physical therapy at a rehabilitation facility. The social worker in charge of her discharge planning, as well as her physician, recommended nursing home placement. Both Mrs. H. and her daughters were unwilling to make this choice if it could be avoided. One of her daughters contacted the local area agency on aging where a case manager was able to put together a package of home health care services that, combined with informal care, allowed Mrs. H. to return home.

Mrs. P: Mrs. P. is a 72-year-old widow who lives alone in an older home located next door to her widowed brother. As a result of an acute health care episode requiring hospitalization, she has difficulty with all ADLs except for eating, and also needs help with grocery shopping, laundry, heavy housework, and meal preparation. Mrs. P. copes with these difficulties through the use of special equipment (e.g., electric bed, shower seat, bedside commode, grab bars) and a mix of formal and informal helpers, including her brother, one of her sons, two friends, and a homemaker aide. Before discharge from the hospital, her physician and a social worker met with Mrs. P., her brother, and her oldest son to discuss care plans. The professionals both recommended that she enter a nursing home, at least on a temporary basis, due to her frail condition. Mrs. P. was opposed to that choice. Her brother's proximity and willingness to stay with her at night for a few weeks made it possible for her to return home. Initially she received over 20 hours of home health care each week, along with a great deal of informal help. She currently receives only six hours of assistance a week from a homemaker aide, as well as help with yard work and transportation from her son and brother.

their ability to remain completely independent. They compared their current status with other levels of independence or dependence they had experienced, or with the status of friends or relatives. Those women who appeared most independent (i.e., self-care) and least independent (i.e., nursing home care) compared themselves only to other women they knew, and always to someone whom they considered less independent. For example, Mrs. W.'s physical function had deteriorated to such an extent that she needed help with most personal care tasks. Like other women who had experienced declines in health, she initially compared her situation to her former state of living independently and recognized that she had lost that independence. But she went on to describe the many activities and events she attended at her nursing home. Describing how much she missed her home and wish she could return there, she concluded, "But I oughtta be happy, 'cause I'm lots better off than some of these people [i.e., other residents]–at least I can get around by myself!" She was referring to her ability to push herself through the halls in her wheelchair, without help from any staff members. Thus, her conceptualization of independence had shifted from absolute independence–caring for herself in her own home, to relative independence–her ability to come and go as she wished within the confines of the home.

Women who received help from formal and/or informal helpers made comparisons both with other women and other conditions they had experienced. Several compared themselves with a friend or acquaintance, usually someone of similar age. For example, Mrs. C., unable to remain in her home alone following hip replacement surgery, chose to move into an apartment in a senior housing complex. While expressing some regret that she can no longer be "on my own," she stated with pride that she can still "make my own decisions." Her conceptualization of independence encompassed the ability to make her own decisions about her daily activities. Mrs. H., the most disabled respondent and the one receiving the most assistance, described how she gets up by herself each morning and fixes her own breakfast. She called attention to her neat home, describing how she had always kept it clean and "shining," even when her daughters were young. "Now I know I can't do the work. . . . My daughters help so I can stay here. It's real hard some days . . . but I'm thankful I'm still living in my own home." She described a former neighbor who had been admitted to a nursing home following a stroke that left her partially paralyzed. Mrs. H. conceptualized independence as avoiding entering a nursing home.

Other participants in the decision process also assigned meaning to independence in relative terms, but their comparisons were inclined to be more fixed. They were also focused on what was lost, rather than on abilities and independence that remained for the older women. Children most often compared their mother's current state, regardless of her level of disability, to the "way she used to be," as one son phrased it, referring to his mother before she had difficulty and was still independent. Children also tended to view their mother's independence relative to her actual need for help and to their participation in helping her. That is, they considered that they were "helping" her and were compelled to recognize her loss of independence primarily when she actually needed *their* assistance. For example, Mrs. P.'s son stated:

> You know, I always stopped up every other week or so to visit, to see my uncle [next door] . . . sometimes we'd work in the garden or mow her lawn and she fixed lunch. Now I have to get there every other week to mow or it just sits there waiting for me.

Another example is Mrs. H.'s daughter, who described a tradition that she and her mother had shared for many years:

> We always go out on Friday . . . to the hairdresser, to the mall for some shopping, usually for lunch. We've done this for years together, almost every week. When we started it was just a fun time together . . . just the girls going out, you know? Now mom needs a lot of help, getting in and out of the car, you know? And I always have to drive.

While the adult children's attention was directed toward the independent end of the continuum and their mothers' movement away from it, service providers tended to focus on the dependent end of the continuum and their efforts to prevent the women's movement toward it. They consistently voiced the desire to avoid nursing home placement for their clients when at all possible and attempted to supply the services necessary to avoid that outcome. Mrs. H.'s case manager, for example, stated:

> I never want to recommend nursing home placement even though it's sometimes the best choice. No one wants to go to a nursing home . . . we have so many more services now, and ways to help people at home . . . if we can just find the right combination of help . . . and there's family, too . . . then we can keep our clients independent.

Concerns About Safety

All participants referred to the conflict between maximizing the older women's independence and still guarding her safety. The issue was discussed more frequently by service providers and the older women themselves, however. While independence and safety are not mutually exclusive, it becomes harder to secure both as people's frailty increases. Mrs. W. and Mrs. C. expressed concerns about their own safety if they continued to live alone. As a result of these fears, each gave up her home to move to a less independent situation. In Mrs. C.'s case, this choice was made in spite of the proximity of a supportive daughter who would have helped her mother to remain in her home. Mrs. H. and Mrs. P. expressed more concern about leaving their homes than they did about being safe alone. Each woman had family members willing and able to help them continue to live in their homes.

Social workers were particularly conflicted when an older woman was very frail. They felt responsible for ensuring that no physical harm came to the older women and were reluctant for them to stay alone in their homes. In the cases of Mrs. H. and Mrs. P., the combination of supportive family members and determined older women overcame the providers' fears about the women living alone. Mrs. H.'s case manager stated clearly that she "could never have agreed to this arrangement if it weren't for her daughters living so close."

The Family's Importance in Maintaining Independence

Case managers described the tension inherent in attempting to protect their client's independence when faced with concerns about safety (e.g., high risk of falling). The fact that their perceived expertise and specialized knowledge of the system often results in an imbalance of decision-making power in their favor adds further complexity to their decision-making process. When weighing these issues, case managers tended to place more value on preserving the client's safety and preferred to choose a more dependent care arrangement when a less dependent arrangement was associated with any real risk. This propensity to reduce client independence was counterbalanced by the intervention of family members who were willing to take responsibility for their older relative's safety, however. On occasion, relevant service providers agreed to a care arrangement that they did not perceive as being safe in order to preserve the woman's perception of independence and to satisfy family's preferences. Mrs. H.'s case is an excellent example. Although extremely disabled and at high risk for injury since she lives alone, her daughters' availability and willingness to help persuaded the relevant professionals to agree to this care arrangement. Her case manager describes the situation:

> I never thought when I first saw Mrs. H. that she would go home . . . [she was] so sick. She could barely get in and out of bed by herself . . . couldn't walk more than a few steps even with a walker. Her daughters were just insisting that she had to go home . . . a nursing home would 'kill her.' But they couldn't give her enough help. We finally put together enough services so that we agreed to try letting her go home . . . So far it's working okay, but if she falls again when she's alone I don't know . . . it's only because of her daughters she can manage now.

Mrs. P.'s case provides another example. Her case manager discussed her reluctance to let Mrs. P. return home after a hospitalization, preferring that she spend some time in a rehabilitation facility.

> She just insisted on going home, wouldn't even consider the rehab placement. I was really worried about her being out there so far from any emergency services. If it wasn't for her brother next door . . . and she promised she'd go to the rehab hospital if her home health nurse recommended it, or else we never would have agreed to let her go home.

Responsibility and Reciprocity

There was clear evidence that the adult children in this study felt a sense of responsibility to provide help in the face of their mothers' frailty. This supports earlier findings that filial concern predicts both instrumental and emotional support (Whitbeck, Hoyt, & Huck, 1994). Conflicting with this sense of responsibility, however, was their preference for maintaining the mother's, as well as their own, independence. This tension underlies Matthews and Rosner's principle of least involvement which functions "to preserve the independence of both generations for as long as possible" (1988, p. 187). For example, following Mrs. C.'s hip replacement she faced two immediate alternatives: return home alone or move in with her daughter. While her daughter was fully prepared to share her home, it was not her preference. "I've got plenty of room for her here, but I'm not sure she'd be happy . . . it has to be her decision." Nor was it Mrs. C.'s preference. "I wanted to go home. . . . I've lived in that house for over 40 years, raised my kids there. [I would] just be on top of them all the time if I go to my daughter's." She did spend a few weeks at her daughter's home before moving to an assisted living facility nearby. Mrs. C.'s daughter feels that her mother is "happier in her own place. We don't get in each other's way now . . . I still see her almost every day so I know she's doing okay."

Previous research shows that assistance given by adult children to parents is often based on the desire to reciprocate for aid and nurturance they have received over their lives (Dwyer, Lee, & Jankowski, 1994). This study supports that notion as well. Many of the adult children interviewed discussed their appreciation for their mother's care when they were young and dependent, and made it clear that they were glad to help now that the situation was reversed. A broader concept of reciprocity emerged from this study, however. Rather than being based solely on reciprocal assistance in a specific parent-child dyad, it recognizes and reciprocates for help given elsewhere. For example, Mrs. H.'s daughter felt that the help she was now giving her mother was a return for her mother's care for her father after his heart attack. Mrs. P. alluded to this as well when she stated that she felt "blessed to get all this help . . . just like I was a blessing to my parents when I took care of them."

DISCUSSION

This qualitative study explored participants' perceptions of the decision-making process associated with various care arrangements for frail older women, most of whom were widows. It makes three contributions to our understanding of how different care arrangements are chosen. First, it identifies the central importance of independence as the basis for decision making, and elucidates the various meanings that care arrangement participants can attach to the term "independence." That is, while all participants might define independence absolutely as the ability to care for oneself, they attributed relative meanings to the term depending on their situation. Independence for the older women is best understood not as some fixed notion, but rather as a flexible concept which each one redefined as her own condition changed. The primary reasons for this were to ensure some self-perceived level of independence, and to help them cope when compelled to adjust to a less independent state. This flexibility in defining independence enabled the older women in this sample to acquiesce and adapt to a care arrangement that they may have needed, but did not necessarily prefer.

Children, on the other hand, tended to have a fixed notion of independence which encompassed their desire for their mothers to be able to take care of themselves if possible and to get at least some of the necessary help elsewhere if not. Once involved in helping in response to a mother's need, the children in this study viewed her as less independent. Alternatively, when her need was met by others (e.g., the service provision system), they were inclined to view her as still somewhat independent in relative, if not absolute, terms. That is, children's perception of a mother's independence can have relative meaning: her independence is compromised when they are involved in helping and when she actually needs that help.

Service providers tended to focus on a narrow view of independence–avoiding nursing home placement. As a result, they often went to great lengths to organize the appropriate home- and community-based services necessary to avoid that outcome.

Second, it would be difficult to overstate the important role that family members play in the care arrangement decision process. Clearly the availability of family members and their participation in both the decision-making process and the eventual care arrangement were crucial factors in several of the decisions. While the inclusion of family members adds complexity to the decision process, their presence can work in favor of those women whom professionals want to place in more dependent care arrangements than the women, or their family members, prefer. Women without family members available to participate in the decision-making process, and particularly in the care arrangement, may be more likely to find themselves living with care arrangement decisions essentially made for them by professionals.

Taken together, these findings have implications for service providers and policymakers. The projected growth in the use of formal long-term care services suggests that providers will continue to be an integral part of many care arrangement decisions. As the recognized "expert" participants, professional service providers wield a great deal of power during the decision-making process. It is important to realize that some older persons may agree to care arrangements they do not necessarily prefer, provided they can maintain a sense of their own independence. This ability to adapt to an outcome they may not have chosen on their own can make them vulnerable to the preferences of other decision makers. In light of this, service providers might want to formulate interventions that will enhance older persons' perceptions of their own independence, or assist individuals who are experiencing difficulty adapting to a given care arrangement. This would be especially appropriate in those care arrangements, such as nursing homes, where the most independence may be sacrificed. The knowledge that older persons will sometimes agree to a care arrangement they do not want should encourage health care professionals, particularly discharge planners, to remain vigilant in protecting their clients' best interests.

A second implication is associated with growth in the use of formal services. We have seen that case managers attempt to ensure their clients' best interests and safety, while adult children prefer to keep a parent as independent as possible while remaining relatively detached from the care process. Taken together, these results suggest the potential for the use of a great deal of formal community care. This notion is supported by research showing that adult children often serve as a bridge to the formal care service system (Bass & Noelker, 1987; Logan & Spitze, 1994). Policymakers are concerned about the recent growth in long-term care expenditures, particularly Medicare home health care expenditures (National Association for Home Care, 1997). Family members provide the bulk of community care to frail older persons. Changes in family structure, such as increases in the number of one-parent households, combined with women's increased participation in the labor force, may reduce adult children's ability or willingness to continue providing large amounts of informal community care. One result could be an increase in the demand for formal community-based services. As the debate over Medicare reform continues, it will be important for policymakers to understand the dynamics involved in care arrangement decisions.

A final contribution of this study is that it broadens our concept of reciprocity. Research has shown that much of the care provided by children is reciprocal in nature (e.g., Dwyer, Lee, & Jankowski, 1994). That is, children and parents are involved in a resource exchange in which children provide their time and help, either in return for resources parents have shared during their lifetime (e.g., shelter, food), or in return for resources currently being shared by parents (e.g., babysitting). The participants in this study attributed a wider meaning to reciprocity, extending it to resource exchange among individuals outside their individual parent-child dyad. Several adult children felt the help they were providing to their mothers was in some sense a return for assistance she had given to other family members, particularly the children's father. Viewed from the older women's perspective, at least one felt that the help she was receiving from family members and friends was a return for the care she had given her own parents in their old age.

This study has investigated the process surrounding the choice of different care arrangements from the perspective of each of the relevant decision participants. Additional research is needed to determine the generalizability of results. We know that care arrangements for similarly disabled older persons of different racial and ethnic backgrounds are often very different than they are for Whites. For example, Blacks are less likely than Whites to use nursing home care and have broader levels of social support that influence their likelihood to use informal care (Burton et al., 1995; Falcone & Broyles, 1994; Salive et al., 1993). Given this knowledge, it would be particularly informative to study how older individuals from other racial and ethnic backgrounds interact to choose a care arrangement. Information such as this would provide important insight at a time when the older population is expected to become increasingly diverse.

We have seen the primary importance of family in the lives of the older women in this study. All but one were widows with children and many had siblings; many of these family members were involved in the women's daily lives in a material way. Thus, though they had lost a life partner and were often living alone, they were not "on their own again," but were instead located in the midst of supportive family networks.

REFERENCES

Bass, D.M. & Noelker, L.S. (1987). The influence of family caregivers on elder's use of in-home services: An expanded conceptual framework. *Journal of Health and Social Behavior, 28*, 184-196.

Bogden, R. & Taylor, S.J. (1975). *Introduction to Qualitative Research Methods: A Phenomenological Approach to the Social Sciences.* New York: John Wiley and Sons.

Burton, L., Kasper, J., Shore, A., Cagney, K., LaVeist, T., Cubbin, C., & German, P. (1995). The structure of informal care: Are there differences by race? *The Gerontologist, 35*, 744-752.

Coulton, C.J., Dunkle, R.E., Haug, M., Chow, J., & Vielhaber, D.P. (1989). Locus of control and decision making for posthospital care. *The Gerontologist, 29*, 627-632.

DeVault, M.L. (1999). *Liberating Method: Feminism and Social Research.* Philadelphia: Temple University Press.

Dwyer, J., Lee, G.R., & Jankowski, T.B. (1994). Reciprocity, elder satisfaction, and caregiver stress and burden: The exchange of aid in the family caregiving relationship. *Journal of Marriage and the Family, 56*, 35-43.

Falcone, D. & Broyles, R. (1994). Access to long-term care: Race as a barrier. *Journal of Health Politics, Policy and Law, 19*, 583-595.

Gonyea, J.G. (1987). The family and dependency: Factors associated with institutional decision-making. *The Journal of Gerontological Social Work, 12*, 61-77.

Hennessy, C.H. (1989). Autonomy and risk: The role of client wishes in community-based long-term care. *The Gerontologist, 29*, 633-639.

High, D.M. (1988). All in the family: Extended autonomy and expectations in surrogate health care decision-making. *The Gerontologist, 28*, 46-51.

High, D.M. & Rowles, G.D. (1995). Nursing home residents, families, and decision making: Toward an understanding of progressive surrogacy. *Journal of Aging Studies, 9*, 101-117.

Horowitz, A. & Shindelman, L.W. (1983). Reciprocity and affection: Past influences on current caregiving. *Journal of Gerontological Social Work, 5*, 5-20.

Jenkins, C.L. (2002). Resource effects on access to care for frail older people. *Journal of Aging & Social Policy, 13* (forthcoming).

Logan, J.R. & Spitze, G. (1994). Informal support and the use of formal services by older Americans. *Journal of Gerontology: Social Sciences, 49*, S25-S34.

Luborsky, M.R. (1994). The identification and analysis of themes and patterns. In *Qualitative Methods in Aging Research*, J.F. Gubrium & A. Sankar, Eds. Thousand Oaks, CA: Sage.

Matthews, S.H. & Rosner, T.T. (1988). Shared filial responsibility: The family as the primary caregiver. *Journal of Marriage and the Family, 50*, 185-195.

Miller, B., McFall, S., & Campbell, R. (1994). Changes in sources of community long-term care among African Americans and white frail older persons. *The Journal of Gerontology: Social Sciences, 49*, S14-S24.

Miner, S. (1995). Racial differences in family support and formal service utilization among older persons: A nonrecursive model. *Journal of Gerontology: Social Sciences, 50B*, S143-S153.

National Association for Home Care. (1997). *Basic Statistics About Home Care 1996*. Washington, DC: National Association for Home Care.

Pratt, C., Jones, L., Shin, H., & Walker, A. (1989). Autonomy and decision-making among single older women and their caregiving daughters. *The Gerontologist, 29*, 792-797.

Prohaska, T.R. & Glasser, M. (1996). Patients' views of family involvement in medical care decisions and encounters. *Research on Aging, 18*, 52-69.

Salive, M.E., Collins, K.S., Foley, D.J., & George, L.K. (1993). Predictors of nursing home admission in a biracial population. *American Journal of Public Health, 83*, 1765-1767.

Wetle, T. (1995). Ethical issues and value conflicts facing case managers of frail elderly people living at home. In *Long-Term Care Decisions: Ethical and Conceptual Dimensions*, L.B. McCullough & N.L. Wilson, Eds. Baltimore, MD: Johns Hopkins University Press.

Wetle, T., Levkoff, S., Cwikel, J., & Rosen, A. (1988). Nursing home resident participation in medical decisions: Perceptions and preferences. *The Gerontologist, 28*, 32-38.

Whitbeck, L., Hoyt, D.R., & Huck, S.M. (1994). Early family relationships, intergenerational solidarity, and support provided to parents by their adult children. *Journal of Gerontology: Social Sciences, 49*, S85-S94.

Widowhood and Spirituality: Coping Responses to Bereavement

Scott T. Michael, PhD
Martha R. Crowther, PhD
Bettina Schmid, MA
Rebecca S. Allen, PhD

SUMMARY. Nearly half of women age 65 or older are widows and nearly 70% of these women live alone. Because older women are three times more likely than their male counterparts to be widowed, widowhood has been labeled a primarily female phenomenon. This review article has two aims: (a) to discuss the impact of widowhood on the lives of older women and (b) to discuss how religion and spirituality may be used as coping methods for conjugal loss. After reviewing the literature the authors conclude that older women use religious coping as well as religious and spiritual beliefs and behaviors to facilitate positive adjustment to the loss of a spouse. *[Article copies available for a fee from The Haworth Document Delivery Service: 1-800-HAWORTH. E-mail address: <docdelivery@ haworthpress.com> Website: <http://www.HaworthPress.com> © 2003 by The Haworth Press, Inc. All rights reserved.]*

Address correspondence to: Martha R. Crowther, PhD, MPH, The University of Alabama Department of Psychology, Box 870348, Tuscaloosa, AL 35487-0348 (E-mail: crowther@bama.ua.edu).

This manuscript was partially supported by The University of Alabama Research Advisory Committee Account No. 2-67709 to R. Allen and The National Institute on Aging Account No. R01 AG 15062-03S1 to M. Crowther.

[Haworth co-indexing entry note]: "Widowhood and Spirituality: Coping Responses to Bereavement." Michael et al. Co-published simultaneously in *Journal of Women & Aging* (The Haworth Press, Inc.) Vol. 15, No. 2/3, 2003, pp. 145-165; and: *Widows and Divorcees in Later Life: On Their Own Again* (ed: Carol L. Jenkins) The Haworth Press, Inc., 2003, pp. 145-165. Single or multiple copies of this article are available for a fee from The Haworth Document Delivery Service [1-800-HAWORTH, 9:00 a.m. - 5:00 p.m. (EST). E-mail address: docdelivery@haworthpress.com].

KEYWORDS. Spirituality, widowhood, religion, coping

Nearly half of women 65 years old or older are widows and nearly 70% of these women live alone (U.S. Census Bureau, 2000). This is partially due to the trend in American society for women to marry older men. Additionally, the average life span for men remains shorter than the average life span for women. Overall, women may live 15 years as widows (Carstensen, 1991).

Because older women are three times more likely than their male counterparts to be widowed, widowhood has been labeled a primarily female phenomenon (Brubaker, 1985). Conjugal bereavement represents the vast majority of the bereavement literature (Nolen-Hoeksema & Larson, 1999). The terms "bereavement" and "grief" are often used interchangeably in the literature. For the purposes of this article, we will adopt the definitions by Marwit (1991) who defined bereavement as "an objective state of having experienced a loss" and grief as "a subjective state of psychological and physiological reaction to that loss" (p. 76).

Bereavement affects many areas of a person's life, including emotional well-being, self-concept, physical health, social relationships, involvement in leisure activities, and religious participation (Lund & Caserta, 1998). People vary considerably in how they respond to the loss of a spouse. Reactions range from transient distress to persistent mental, emotional, and/or physical problems (Stroebe & Stroebe, 1993). In this article, we will review the literature on issues that impact the bereavement experience of older women and how spirituality and religious coping may facilitate positive adjustment.

ISSUES THAT IMPACT THE EXPERIENCE OF WIDOWHOOD

Adjustment to widowhood is related to several factors, including: (a) the bereaved person's age and the circumstances that surround the loved one's death, (b) caregiving experiences, (c) psychological distress, (d) physical health problems, (e) current social support, and (f) the use of terminal care services.

Age and the timing of death. In general, younger widowhood has been associated with a greater risk for negative outcomes (Stroebe & Stroebe, 1987). When the spousal death occurs "off time"–at an unexpected stage in life (Seltzer, 1976) or suddenly (Lemme, 2002), the surviving spouse is thrust into widowhood with little preparation and often experiences more stress than women who lose a spouse at an expected life stage or as a result of a prolonged illness. Additionally, financial trouble may ensue as a result of a decrease in income after spousal death and limited earning capacity among older women (Troll, 1986; Lemme, 2002). This effect is magnified among minority women whose husbands die at a younger age and whose families tend to have lower financial status (Lemme, 2002).

How do older widows differ from their younger counterparts? Are there special issues that older widows tend to experience because of their age? One of the unique issues facing older widows is ageism and how ageist beliefs impact both younger persons' perspectives as well as the perspectives of older adults themselves. For example, Moss, Moss, and Hansson (2001), point out that older adults may feel a pressure, both internally and externally, to suppress their grief. In an ageist culture, older persons displaying grief may be viewed as unseemly or, perhaps worse, unnecessary. If the deceased family member was elderly, it may be viewed within the family system as being "time" for the person to go, thus intense grief is viewed as excessive. Additionally, younger family members may be the focal point of grieving within the family unit, and thus the older adult may be relegated to a peripheral grieving role. Cultural beliefs tend to downplay the "tragedy" of an older person's death, which may leave the older widow to grieve alone, especially after the initial ceremonies of mourning (e.g., rosaries, wakes, funerals).

Older widows often have other challenges related to current societal standards and social structures. Adults tend to focus their social networks as they age on more fulfilling relationships (Carstensen, Gross, & Fung, 1997). Thus, the impact of bereavement may lead to greater vulnerability given the loss of a primary social support. Also, they may be forced to relocate by family members who live in other places, thus losing other important social support (Moss et al., 2001).

There have been several studies that have compared older and younger widows. The acute phase of bereavement may be less distressing for older widows (Sanders, 1993). Older widows, however, may experience a slower decline in grief symptoms than do younger widows (Sanders, 1981; Thompson et al., 1991). Mendes de Leon, Kasl, and Jacobs (1994) found that depression often persists past the first year post-bereavement for the younger elderly widows (65 years to 74 years) but not for the older widows (over 75 years). The latter result may seem to contradict the former, but perhaps there are differential effects for younger versus older widows, depending on the researcher's definition of "older." Some studies examined women 54 and older (Carnelley, Wortman, & Kessler, 1999) whereas others sampled women over the age of 75 years (Mendes de Leon et al., 1994). With the steadily growing population of older women and the lengthening of average life spans, future research should make distinctions in the young-old (age 65 to 74), the old-old (age 75 to 80) and the oldest-old (over 80 years).

Caregiving. Prior experience as a caregiver to the deceased also impacts a woman's adjustment to bereavement. In a study of elderly spouses, Schultz et al. (2001) found that adjustment to bereavement varies according to the level of strain the bereaved individual experienced prior to the death of the spouse. Specifically, caregivers who reported strain associated with caregiving experienced high levels of depression that remained stable after the death of the patient. Additionally, strained caregivers reported an increase in their performance of positive health behaviors after the spouse's death, whereas non-strained caregivers and non-caregivers exhibited no change in the frequency of their performance of positive health behaviors. At the same time, non-caregivers suffered a significant reduction in weight after bereavement, while those in the caregiving groups did not experience significant weight change.

In a 3-year prospective study of women aged 54 or older, Carnelley and colleagues (1999) found that women whose husbands were ill at baseline did not report significant increases in depression at follow-up. Their baseline levels of depression, however, were elevated at the initial data collection. In contrast, Wyatt, Friedman, Given, and Given (1999) described bereaved spousal caregivers (75% women) of terminally ill patients as suffering from above average levels of depression at three months. Wheaton (1990) found that participants who viewed their marriage as a chronic stressor (e.g., due to chronic illness or bad marriage) reported increased well-being following the death of their spouse.

Psychological well-being. Psychological well-being may be greatly impacted by the death of a spouse. Depression is a common outcome of bereavement for older adults. Jacobs (1993) noted that up to one-third of people experience detrimental effects on their mental and/or physical health after the death of a close family member, and a quarter of widows and widowers suffer from depression and anxiety during the first year of bereavement. Zisook and Shuchter (1993) found that, in a sample of older bereaved adults (71% of whom were women), the prevalence of depression was quite high. Within two months following conjugal bereavement, 24% met criteria for major depression, as compared to 4%

of a married comparison group. This percentage decreased to 14% at 2-year follow-up, which remained significantly greater than the non-bereaved comparison group. In the bereaved sample, major depression was associated with poorer physical health, relationship difficulties, and poorer role functioning.

Physical health. Health problems are another important dimension of adjustment. Schaefer and colleagues (Schafer, Quesenberry, & Wi, 1995) found that mortality following spousal bereavement was elevated even after adjusting for age, education, and comorbid illness. This was particularly true during the first seven to twelve months. However, other research indicates that older widows suffer fewer health consequences of bereavement, especially with regard to mortality (Stroebe & Schut, 2001). The relationship between age of the bereaved person and mortality/morbidity rates appears to be curvilinear, with middle-aged widows suffering higher mortality and morbidity rates than either younger or older widows. Stroebe and Schut suggest that this may be due to the nature of death in middle-aged spouses (i.e., sudden), as compared to death following protracted illness in older spouses. However, there are no well-controlled published studies at the present time to support this hypothesis.

Social support. Several studies have shown that widows have an extensive social support network that helps them cope with the loss of their spouse (Anderson, 1984; Atchley, Pignatiello, & Shae, 1975; Brubaker, 1985). Social support from family and friends has been shown to help the bereaved person go through the grief process with improved psychological well-being (Kaunonen, Tarkka, Paunonen, & Laippala, 1999; Nolen-Hoeksema & Larson, 1999; Sanders, 1993; Stroebe & Stroebe, 1987). Widows apparently perceive their social support to be good relative to both widowers and other bereaved family members. In their prospective study of bereaved individuals recruited through hospices, Nolen-Hoeksema and Larson (1999) found that spouses reported feeling more supported immediately following the death than other family members, perhaps because family members rallied to provide support and care to the spouse. However, as stated earlier, prolonged grief may be viewed negatively and subsequently they receive less support over time (Moss, Moss, & Hansson, 2001).

Utilization of terminal care services. Use of terminal services also has been found to impact adjustment to bereavement. Kelly et al. (1999) found that the severity of the patient's illness at the time of referral to palliative care is a risk factor for adverse bereavement outcomes. McCorkle and colleagues (McCorkle, Robinson, Nuamah, Lev, &

Benoliel, 1998) found that intensive nursing care during the terminal phase of the patient's illness was associated with less psychological distress for spouses following bereavement. However, length of use of terminal services may impact adjustment to bereavement. Gilbar (1998) found that a short length of stay in hospice care (up to one week) had a beneficial effect for bereaved spouses in comparison with hospice stays lasting longer than one week.

The impact of bereavement and grief on the lives of older women and the relative effects of spirituality and religious coping on these normative life events is a phenomenon of growing research interest. Although many factors have been investigated that contribute to widows' adaptive adjustment to their new role, spirituality has often been neglected as a potential coping mechanism used by older women to cope with the loss of their spouse. Older adults are more likely than any other cohort to express religious and spiritual beliefs and practices (McFadden, 1996). Thus, it seems odd that religion and spirituality have been overlooked as potential coping mechanisms in the widowhood literature.

SPIRITUALITY, RELIGION, RELIGIOUS COPING, AND BEREAVEMENT

Definitions

Prior to discussing the role religion, religious coping, and spirituality can play in the lives of widows it is necessary to define the constructs. Part of the problem with incorporating spirituality into the literature has been the confusion associated with the terms religion and spirituality (Krause, 1993). In support of this clarification, we utilize definitions offered by Koenig, McCullough, and Larson (2001): "Religion is an organized system of beliefs, practices, rituals and symbols designed (a) to facilitate closeness to the sacred or transcendent (God, higher power, or ultimate truth/reality), and (b) to foster an understanding of one's relation and responsibility to others in living together in a community" (p. 18). In contrast, "spirituality is the personal quest for understanding answers to ultimate questions about life, about meaning, and about relationship to the sacred or transcendent, which may (or may not) lead to or arise from the development of religious rituals and the formation of community" (p. 18). Pargament (1997) has contributed to our understanding of how religious coping differs from religious beliefs. Religious coping is defined as, "the use of religious beliefs or behaviors to facilitate problem-solving to prevent or alleviate the negative emotional consequences of stressful life circumstances" (p. 513; Koenig, Pargament, & Nielsen, 1998). Pargament (1997) uses the term religious orientations to describe frameworks of beliefs, or frames of reference, which guide behavior in stressful times. Religious coping acts as a "bridge" between religious orientations and the emotional and behavioral outcomes of negative life events. Religious orientations are macro-level schema whereas religious coping strategies are situation-specific methods that mediate the relationship between orientations and outcomes, that is, what someone actually does with these frameworks to deal with stressors. Religious coping predicts psychosocial outcome better than general measures of religiousness (for a review, see Pargament, 1997), supporting the notion that religious coping contributes unique information from religious beliefs.

Increasingly, there is discussion in the literature regarding the relation between religion and spirituality. Some regard the constructs as indistinguishable, while others argue that religion and spirituality are uniquely different with religion referring to a group activity that involves specific behavioral, social, doctrinal, and denominational characteristics (Abeles et al., 1999) and spirituality referring to a personal search for answers regarding life, meaning and relationship to the sacred or transcendent (Koenig, McCullogh, & Larson, 2001). We posit that religion and spirituality can each foster the development of the other. For example, religious practices encourage spiritual growth, while spiritual practices are often a salient aspect of religious participation (Armstrong & Crowther, 2002). Given that many older adults indicate that religion is very important to them (Princeton Religious Research Center, 1994) and persons working with older adults in applied settings have expressed a need for interventions to include a spiritual component (McFadden, 1996), we think it is important to discuss both religion and spirituality and how those factors influence coping in older widows.

In the next section, we will initially examine the role that religious coping plays in facilitating adaptive adjustment to a major life stressor such as conjugal bereavement. Then, we will focus on three modes by which religious coping may aid in the bereavement process: (a) religious coping as meaning construction, (b) religious coping as acquisition of social support and (c) the use of spiritual beliefs as a means of maintaining connections to the deceased.

RELIGIOUS COPING AND ADJUSTMENT
TO BEREAVEMENT AND OTHER MAJOR LIFE STRESSORS

A few studies have found that for many people, religious coping and reliance on religious/spiritual beliefs often are important aspects of responding to difficult life experiences. In a community-based sample, faith was the second most frequently cited coping strategy for dealing with events categorized as threats and third for strategies dealing with loss (McCrae, 1984). Bulman and Wortman (1977) reported that individuals paralyzed in an accident cited God's plan most often as a reason for the accident. Koenig, George, and Siegler (1988) sampled older adults about their coping strategies in the face of stressful life events. The most frequent response was religious coping, reported by forty-five percent of the sample. Clearly, religious coping is a vital aspect of how many individuals respond to painful and stressful events.

According to some religious coping theorists (Koenig et al., 1998; Pargament, Ensing, Falgout, Olsen, Reilly, Van Haitsma, & Warren, 1990; Pargament, 1997; Pargament, Koenig, & Perez, 2000; Pargament, Olsen, Reilly, Falgout, Ensing, & Van Haitsma, 1992; Pargament, Smith, Koenig, & Perez, 1998), religious coping is conceptualized as an active, effortful approach to decrease negative affect and increase psychological well-being. Based on this conceptualization, Pargament, Koenig and Perez (2000) developed a religious coping scale (RCOPE) to assess the full range of religious coping methods, including both adaptive as well as maladaptive religious coping strategies. While many other researchers have theorized religious coping as either adaptive or maladaptive, a comprehensive theory of religious coping should be multidimensional and incorporate the many ways in which people use their spiritual/religious beliefs in response to life events.

In an attempt to determine the unique contribution of religious coping instruments, Pargament (1997) reviewed the coping literature and found several studies that demonstrate the unique predictive power of religious coping as compared to non-religious coping measures. Additionally, Pargament and his colleagues have found that religious coping is a stronger predictor of psychological well-being following a major stressor than more general measures of religiousness (for a review, see Pargament, 1997).

Research shows that older adults benefit from religious coping (Koenig et al., 1998). In a study of older adults hospitalized for serious illnesses, positive religious coping variables such as reappraisal of God as benevolent, collaboration with God, seeking a connection with God, seeking support from clergy/members, and giving religious help to others predicted elevated well-being (Koenig et al., 1998). Interestingly, poorer health was associated with both positive and negative religious coping variables (such as punishing God reappraisals, spiritual discontent, and pleading for direct intercession). The authors hypothesize that graver illnesses may mobilize the use of religious coping strategies; however, for those who use more negative religious coping strategies, they suffer poorer health outcomes. This study points to the adaptive nature of positive religious coping for older adults facing major life stressors.

It is important to note that the RCOPE and the variables in other studies often use a Christian-based, or other supreme being-based, conceptualization of religious coping. For example, many of the items in the RCOPE refer to "God," and the samples used to validate the measure were predominately Christian (Pargament et al., 2000). Given the demographics of the United States, with a high percentage of the population stating a Christian religious affiliation, these studies may be viewed as fairly representative of the population; however, the use of non-Christian oriented spiritual beliefs in coping with stressors should not be ignored. Unfortunately, there is a paucity of research on non-Christian measures.

Religious Coping and Bereavement

Reasonably, we can assume that religious coping, for religiously or spiritually oriented people, can be a crucial aspect of moving through the grieving process, and it is no surprise to learn that the research supports this assumption. A number of studies have found significant associations between religious beliefs/religious coping and adaptive bereavement (Glick, Weiss, & Parkes, 1974; McIntosh, Silver, & Wortman, 1993; Nolen-Hoeksema & Larson, 1999; Park & Cohen, 1993). For example, widows of the Sunshine Mine fire who reported religious beliefs and church involvement judged their quality of life to be more stable five years following their loss as compared to those widows who did not endorse religious beliefs and church involvement (Bahr & Harvey, 1979). In another study, religious/spiritual beliefs were significantly correlated with positive affect for bereaved respondents (Richards & Folkman, 1997). Taken together, these studies give support to the benefit of religious beliefs and religious coping in the grief process. There are likely to be a number of ways that religious coping aids bereaved older women, but we will focus on three major domains of adaptation to bereavement that may best explain the function religious coping has in bereavement.

Religious coping as meaning construction. Over the past several decades, some studies have found a positive association between finding meaning and adapting to bereavement (Bower, Kemeny, Taylor, & Fahey, 1998; Davis, Nolen-Hoeksema, & Larson, 1998; Moskowitz, Folkman, Collette, & Vittinghoff, 1996; Stein, Folkman, Trabasso, & Richards, 1997). In a study of HIV-positive men who lost a loved one to AIDS-related causes, Bower and her colleagues (1998) found that finding meaning predicted slower rates of CD4 T cell decline, a marker of poor health for HIV-positive individuals, and less mortality. Similarly, Moskowitz et al. (1996) reported that positive reappraisals of the experience of the death of a loved one due to AIDS-related diseases was associated with increased positive affect. These studies point to the positive role that finding meaning has in the grieving process. Moreover, McIntosh et al. (1993) reported that religious beliefs were associated with finding meaning in the death of an infant. Thus, religious beliefs may facilitate finding meaning as a coping strategy.

In a study of older adults asked to focus on their most negative life event (including the death of a loved one), Tait and Silver (1989) found that ongoing cognitive and emotional involvement in the event, including trying to find a meaningful perspective, were related to lessened quality of life and self-assessed recovery from the event. The average length of time since the negative event was approximately 23 years. This study suggests that ongoing searches for meaning in painful experiences may be a disruptive, distressing process when no adequate meaning may be found. Tait and Silver (1989) hypothesize that painful life events may motivate a meaning-search process that continues, perhaps in the form of painful and intrusive rumination, until sufficient meaning is found, or constructed. Thus, those who have difficulty finding satisfactory meaning may continue to suffer from the pain that arises from a lack of resolution.

Meaning is, itself, a multidimensional concept, and the meanings individuals find in experiences such as bereavement are likely to vary greatly. Some attempts, however, have been made to categorize construals of meaning in order to better understand the role meaning construction has in adjustment to painful/traumatic life events. Making sense of the death concerns understanding the death in the context of one's world beliefs, whereas benefit finding concerns construing positive outcomes from the experience. Affleck and Tennen (1996) have written extensively on the adaptive nature of benefit finding in coping with major stressors. This concept also has been termed posttraumatic growth (Tedeschi & Calhoun,

1996), positive reinterpretation (Scheier, Weintraub, & Carver, 1986), and stress-related growth (Park, Cohen, & Murch, 1996).

Using the distinction in construals of meaning proposed by Janoff-Bulman and Frantz (1997), Davis and colleagues (1998) examined the roles that making sense of the death and finding some benefit in the death had in the bereavement process. The respondents in this study were recruited through hospices while their loved ones were still living, were initially interviewed at that time, and were re-interviewed at 1-month, 6-month, 13-month, and 18-month follow-up post-loss. Davis et al. (1998) found that making sense of the death was predictive of positive adjustment within the first year following the death, while finding benefits was a better predictor at the 13-month and 18-month follow-up interviews. The authors theorize that there are different processes involved in the search for each construal of meaning that explain the differences. Making sense of the death may be initially important when one's worldview has been disrupted by the death (see Janoff-Bulman, 1992). We have a need to maintain a coherent framework for understanding the world and our place in it and this need motivates a process to re-establish this framework when it has been disrupted. On the other hand, finding benefits in bereavement may be part of a positive reframing coping strategy that takes time to unfold and have its beneficial impact on the bereaved individual's life.

It is reasonable that belief systems that can assimilate the occurrence of death within their frameworks would be less disrupted and allow for a more facile sense-making process. Spiritual/religious beliefs may be such systems. Indeed, Davis et al. (1998) found that such beliefs pre-loss were predictive of later sense-making. Alternatively, spiritual/religious beliefs did not predict finding benefits.

Other research has supported the connection between religious coping and finding meaning in adversity. In the Koenig et al. (1998) study of older adults with serious illnesses, some positive religious coping variables had a stronger association with stress-related growth than non-religious coping variables. This suggests that religious coping is an important aspect of finding benefits in very stressful life events. The religious coping strategies with the strongest correlation to stress-related growth were seeking a spiritual connection to God, collaborative coping with God, seeking support from clergy or church members, and benevolent reappraisals of God. Bear in mind that the Davis et al. (1998) study looked at religious beliefs whereas the Koenig et al. (1998) study focused more specifically on religious coping. Perhaps the religious coping strategies mentioned above have a unique relationship to finding meaning in comparison with general religious beliefs.

It may be that spiritual/religious beliefs, themselves, offer a framework for comprehending the "why" of a loved one's death. They provide the bereaved acceptable answers in their search to explain the loss in the scheme of things. An older woman who recently lost her spouse of many years will very likely turn to her beliefs in her search to make sense of her devastating loss. If she has a pre-established system of spiritual belief that offers a ready-made explanation of the death and places it in a higher framework of meaning (e.g., "it is God's will and I will rejoin my partner in the afterlife"), she is likely to find more comfort and sense of well-being than a widow who feels devoid of such explanations.

Religious coping as acquisition of social support. As Nolen-Hoeksema and Larson (1999) discuss, the nature of social networks has changed a great deal in contemporary times. Previously, the majority of a recently widowed woman's family lived around her and she was likely to be an integral member of a community she had lived in her whole life. With the modernization of our culture, families are often spread throughout the country and many persons have moved multiple times. A recently widowed older woman may be faced, suddenly, with the loss of the majority of her social support, particularly if a number of her other family members live far away. In situations like these, religious communities may offer critical support to the widow. Even in situations where the widow lives near family and in a tightly knit community, her congregation may have been an ongoing source of social support that now is very important to her as she begins to adjust to a new life without her spouse. In the Nolen-Hoeksema and Larson (1999) hospice study, religious/spiritual beliefs were related to stronger social support. People who endorsed having such beliefs and also reported greater religious services attendance experienced stronger social support, less social isolation, and less social friction than those who reported low or no attendance.

Another important element of the support that comes from religious coping is the support of God (or another spiritual presence for other systems of belief). Indeed, this type of support aids many individuals in difficult times (Pargament, 1997). As one woman in the Nolen-Hoeksema and Larson (1999) study stated: My faith has given me everything I need to cope with it. That's why I don't need support groups. I have the greatest support group–God (p. 75).

Pargament (1997) found evidence for the beneficial effects of perceived support from God. Furthermore, collaborative coping with God has often been predictive of positive adjustment to stressors (Pargament, 1997). Collaboration with God would seem to involve a perception that God is an active partner in solving problems in stressful situations, which is certainly viewed as a supportive process.

Moreover, providing support to others may be adaptive. Religious helping has been associated with positive adjustment in medically ill, hospitalized adults (Koenig et al., 1998). In a prospective study of community-dwelling older adults, Oman, Thoresen, and McMahon (1999) found that volunteerism predicted lower mortality rates, even when controlling for potentially confounding factors such as health status (i.e., unable to volunteer due to health problems). This effect was found to be especially protective for respondents reporting higher levels of religious involvement. Thus, providing support via helping behavior leads to positive outcomes for older adults. Although there was no reported evidence that helping behavior is adaptive in times of bereavement, some individuals may benefit from offering others help and support during their own painful times. This may provide the widow with an opportunity to connect with others and, in line with many spiritual beliefs, act in accordance with a moral directive (i.e., help others).

Religious coping as maintaining a bond to the deceased. A less researched area, but no less conceptually interesting, is the use of spiritual beliefs and religious coping to maintain a connection to the lost loved one. This process of "keeping the loved one alive" via conceptualizing him as a spiritual presence and/or as residing in an afterlife state that she can join with some day may be properly viewed as a type of meaning construction, but we wanted to treat this topic separately due to its interesting conceptual nature and the fact that there is little research in this area to date. Many of the meaning finding studies discussed above ask respondents if they have found some meaning in the bereavement experience, and certainly some individuals were responding to this maintained bond as a type of meaning found. These studies do not treat this as a unique type of meaning that either may or may not facilitate adaptive coping with bereavement, however. Some research indicates that non-acceptance of the death is maladaptive (Prigerson et al., 1996; Prigerson et al., 1995), while other studies show that establishing a new identity separate from that of "wife" is an important step for widows in the process of moving through grief (Lopata, 1973). As Worden (1991) states in his seminal book on grief therapy, one of the tasks of bereavement is relocating the emotional bond with the deceased loved one so that bonds with living loved ones may be more of a focus of the bereaved individual's interpersonal life. So, does maintaining a bond with the deceased via spiritual/religious beliefs help or hinder the older widow?

As Stroebe, Gergen, Gergen, and Stroebe (1992) point out, the idea of relocating or "breaking" the bond with the deceased and moving on with one's life is a thoroughly modern idea. The "Grief Work" hypothesis (Stroebe, 1992) that guides much of contemporary bereavement research often holds, as one of its tenets, that adaptive adjustment to grief involves a process of pain as one grieves the deceased, and then a severing of the bond as the bereaved "moves on" with life. On the issue of grief, Freud (1917) spoke of the importance of detaching from a "non-existent" object. In attachment theory, adaptive bereavement is thought to involve a process of detaching from the deceased (Bowlby, 1980). And yet, a growing body of research suggests that maintaining bonds with the deceased is not unhealthy (Klass & Walter, 2001; Stroebe et al., 1992).

As Stroebe et al. (1992) contend, severing the bond with the deceased is a culturally-constructed idea and should be recognized as such. Cross-culturally and at different times within American society varied views have existed regarding the necessity of detaching from the deceased loved one. In a number of cultures, widowhood becomes an identity in and of itself, and the widow is likely to symbolically represent her continued bond with her deceased husband (e.g., wear black, have devotional alters at home).

Spiritual and religious beliefs offer a framework of meaning that explains the tenability of an ongoing presence with which to maintain a bond. The widow's belief system may offer a way of understanding how such a bond can be maintained. It is likely that different types of maintained attachments are more adaptive than others. For example, speaking to a deceased husband during stressful experiences may be comforting. Refusing to accept his death and spending extensive periods of time trying to communicate with him, while neglecting other relationships, may be maladaptive.

FUTURE DIRECTIONS

This article reviewed issues related to widowhood and spirituality. The review suggests that widowhood is an important area of research given the increasing number of widows. Additionally, there are several factors that impact widowhood, including age and timing of death, caregiving experiences, psychological distress, physical health problems, social support, and the use of terminal care services. Also, religious and spiritual beliefs are important components of coping for the current cohort of older widows. It is our hope that the widowhood literature will continue to grow and include prospective studies that focus on adjustment to bereavement among older widows and the role of spirituality. Suggestions for future research directions are described below.

Directions for future research should explore the loss of a partner in same-sex unions. Although we tend to conceptualize widowhood as it refers to heterosexual relationships, there are a minority of older women who have been in long-term homosexual relationships. They deal with many of the same issues as their heterosexual counterparts but often without public acceptance of their role as significant other (Huyck, 1995). The lack of acknowledgement of long-term homosexual relationships among older women can have deleterious effects on their health and well-being. Older lesbians often receive limited support from family and friends. Additionally, they are frequently not recognized in a legal or financial capacity (Huyck, 1995). Thus, they do not receive spousal benefits. In many instances, they are excluded from end-of-life planning for their partner, including such issues as finances, health care, modifications in living arrangements, and funeral plans. They are often an overlooked and undersupported group of bereaved individuals (Lemme, 2002). With regard to spirituality and religion, many religious belief systems do not accept homosexual practices. Thus, these women often receive limited instrumental and emotional support from religious persons and/or communities.

Allen, DeLaine, Chaplin, Marson, Bourgeois, Dijkstra and Burgio (under review) found that the familial proxies of nursing home residents with stronger religiosity were *less* likely to engage in advance care planning for their relatives. This unexpected result corresponds to the finding of Sonnenblick, Friedlander, and Steinberg (1993) that adult children who expressed a higher degree of religiosity and greater closeness in their relationship with a terminally ill parent typically requested continuation or initiation of life-sustaining treatments, even if it meant not complying with parental wishes. Religiosity may play different roles in the end-of-life medical treatment decisions of older adults and their potential proxy decision makers. Further research addressing religiosity and spirituality in the context of familial advance planning (Allen & Shuster, 2002) is needed.

Future studies in the area of religious coping should branch out to include non-Christian/supreme being based spiritual practices. We argue that simply removing Christian terms from instruments (e.g., change from God to higher being) is not sufficient but rather suggest designing instruments that address the unique religious or spiritual belief system of a particular group. Surely such non-traditional methods can be helpful and account for important variance in research results, and yet may be missed by measures that focus on "Christianity." It is important to understand how other religious/spiritual belief systems and practices (e.g., the use of Buddhist meditation as a coping technique) facilitate adaptive coping to stressful life events such as bereavement.

Patterns of bereavement for widows should also be explored, as the "baby boomer" generation becomes the next wave of older adults. Generational differences in coping strategies may change our current understanding of how older widows adapt to the death of a partner. It also will be important to consider the effects of an ever growing population of "oldest-old" (80+ years) adults. As discussed earlier, the oldest-old may cope with bereavement in a much different way than the young-old. Well-designed prospective studies are needed to follow the changes in patterns of adjustment to bereavement for the baby boomers as well as the oldest-old. The patterns of religious coping may change as well. With an increased focus on spirituality (Crowther, Parker, Larimore, Achenbaum, & Koenig, 2002), the role of religious coping in bereavement may change. Finally, research examining the benefit older widows receive from helping others as they adjust to the loss of their spouse may be a fruitful area of investigation.

REFERENCES

Abeles, R., Ellison, C., George, L., Idler, E., Krause, N., Levin, J., Ory, M., Pargament, K., Powell, L., Underwood, L., & Williams, D. (1999). *Multidimensional measurement of religiousness/spirituality for use in health research*. Kalamazoo, MI: Fetzer Institute Publication.

Affleck, G., & Tennen, H. (1996). Construing benefits from adversity: Adaptational significance and dispositional underpinnings. *Journal of Personality, 64*, 899-922.

Allen, R. S., & Shuster, J. L. (2002). The role of proxies in treatment decisions: Evaluating functional capacity to consent to end-of-life treatments within a family context. *Behavioral Sciences and the Law, 20*, 235-252.

Allen, R. S., DeLaine, S., Chaplin, W. F., Marson, D. L., Bourgeois, M., Dijkstra, K., & Burgio, L. D. (under review). Advance care planning in nursing homes: The role of proxy beliefs and resident behavior. Manuscript submitted for publication.

Anderson, T. B. (1984). Widowhood as a life transition: Its impact on Kinship ties. *Journal of Marriage and the Family, 46*, 105-114.

Armstrong, T., & Crowther, M. (2002). Spirituality among older African Americans. *Journal of Adult Development, 9*, 3-12.

Atchley, R., Pignatiello, L., & Shae, E. (1975). *The effect of marital status on social interaction patterns of older women.* Oxford, OH: Scripps Foundation.

Bower, J. E., Kemeny, M. E., Taylor, S. E., & Fahey, J. L. (1998). Cognitive processing, discovery of meaning, CD4 decline, and AIDS-related mortality among bereaved HIV-seropositive men. *Journal of Consulting and Clinical Psychology, 66,* 979-986.

Bowlby, J. (1980). Attachment and loss. Vol. 3. Loss: Sadness and depression. London: Hogarth.

Brubaker, T. (1985). *Later life families.* Beverly Hills, CA: Sage.

Bulman, J., & Wortman, C. (1977). Attributions of blame and coping in the "real world": Severe accident victims react to their lot. *Journal of Personality and Social Psychology, 35,* 351-363.

Carnelley, K. B., Wortman, C. B., & Kessler, R. C. (1999). The impact of widowhood on depression: Findings from a prospective survey. *Psychological Medicine, 29,* 1111-1123.

Carstensen, L. L. (1991). Socioemotional selectivity theory: Social activity in life-span context. In K.W. Schaie & M. P. Lawton (Eds.), *Annual Review of Gerontology and Geriatrics* (Vol. 11, pp. 195-217). New York: Springer.

Carstensen, L. L., Gross, J. J., & Fung, H. H. (1997). The social context of emotional experience. *Annual Review of Gerontology and Geriatrics, 17,* 325-352.

Crowther, M., Parker, M., Larimore, W., Achenbaum, A., & Koenig, H. (2002). Rowe and Kahn's model of successful aging revisited: Spirituality the missing construct. *The Gerontologist, 42, 613-620.*

Davis, C. G., Nolen-Hoeksema, S., & Larson, J. (1998). Making sense of loss and benefiting from the experience: Two construals of meaning. *Journal of Personality and Social Psychology, 75,* 561-574.

Freud, S. (1917). Mourning and melancholia. In J. Starchey (Ed.), *Standard edition of the complete work of Sigmund Freud.* London: Hogarth Press.

Gilbar, O. (1998). Length of cancer patients' stay at a hospice: Does it affect psychological adjustment to the loss of the spouse? *Journal of Palliative Care, 14,* 16-20.

Glick, I., Weiss, R. S., & Parkes, C. M. (1974). *The first year of bereavement.* New York: Wiley.

Huyck, M. H. (1995). Marriage and close relationships of the marital kind. In R. Blieszner & V. H. Bedford (Eds.), *Handbook of aging and the family* (pp.181-200). Westport, CT: Greenwood Press.

Jacobs, S. (1993). *Pathologic grief: Maladaptation to loss.* Washington, DC: American Psychiatric Press.

Janoff-Bulman, R. (1992). *Shattered assumptions: Towards a new psychology of trauma.* New York: Free Press.

Janoff-Bulman, R., & Frantz, C. M. (1997). The impact of trauma on meaning: From meaningless world to meaningful life. In M. Power & C. R. Brewin (Eds.), *The transformation of meaning in psychological therapies* (pp. 91-106). New York: Wiley.

Kaunonen, M., Tarkka, M. T., Paunonen, M., & Laippala, P. (1999). Grief and social support after the death of a spouse. *Journal of Advanced Nursing, 30,* 1304-1311.

Kelly, B., Edwards, P., Synott, R., Neil, C., Baillie, R., & Battistutta, D. (1999). Predictors of bereavement outcome for family carers of cancer patients. *Psychooncology, 8,* 237-249.

Klass, D., & Walter, T. (2001). Processes of grieving: How bonds are continued. In M. S. Stroebe, R. O. Hansson, W. Stroebe, & H. Schut (Eds.), *Handbook of bereavement research: Consequences, coping, and care* (pp. 431-448). Washington, DC: American Psychological Association.

Koenig, H. G., George, L. K., & Siegler, I. C. (1988). The use of religion and other emotion-regulating coping strategies among older adults. *The Gerontologist, 28,* 303-310.

Koenig, H. G., McCullogh, M., & Larson, D. B. (2001). *Handbook of religion and health.* New York: Oxford University Press.

Koenig, H. G., Pargament, K. I., & Nielsen, J. (1998). Religious coping and health status in medically ill hospitalized older adults. *The Journal of Nervous and Mental Disease, 186,* 513-521.

Krause, N. (1993). Measuring religiosity in later life. *Research on Aging, 15,* 170-197.

Lemme, B. H. (2002). *Development in adulthood* (3rd Edition). Needham Heights, MA: Allyn and Bacon.

Lopata, H. (1973). Widowhood in an American city. Morrison, NJ: General Learning Press.

Lund, D. A., & Caserta, M. S. (1998). Future directions in adult bereavement research. *Omega, 36,* 287-303.

Marwit, S. J. (1991). DSM-III-R, grief reactions, and a call for revision. *Professional Psychology: Research and Practice, 22,* 75-79.

McCorkle, R., Robinson, L., Nuamah, I., Lev, E., & Benoliel, J. Q. (1998). The effects of home nursing care for patients during terminal illness on the bereaved's psychological distress. *Nursing Research, 47,* 2-10.

McCrae, R. R. (1984). Situational determinants of coping response: Loss, threat, and challenge. *Journal of Personality and Social Psychology, 46,* 919-928.

McFadden, S. H. (1996). Religion, spirituality, and aging. In J. E. Birren & K. W. Schaie (Eds.) pp. 162-177. *Handbook of the psychology of aging (4th ed.): The handbook of aging.* San Diego, CA: Academic Press, Inc.

McIntosh, D. N., Silver, R. C., & Wortman, C. B. (1993). Religion's role in adjustment to a negative life event: Coping with the loss of a child. *Journal of Personality and Social Psychology, 65,* 812-821.

Mendes de Leon, C. F., Kasl, S. V., & Jacobs, S. (1994). A prospective study of widowhood and changes in symptoms of depression in a community sample of the elderly. *Psychological Medicine, 24,* 613-624.

Moskowitz, J. T., Folkman, S., Collette, L., & Vittinghoff, E. (1996). Coping and mood during AIDS-related caregiving and bereavement. *Annals of Behavioral Medicine, 18,* 49-57.

Moss, M. S., Moss, S. Z., & Hansson, R. O. (2001). Bereavement and old age. In M. S. Stroebe, R. O. Hansson, W. Stroebe, & H. Schut (Eds.), *Handbook of bereavement research: Consequences, coping, and care* (pp. 241-260). Washington, DC: American Psychological Association.

Nolen-Hoeksema, S., & Larson, J. (1999). *Coping with loss.* Mahwah, NJ: Lawrence Erlbaum Associates.

Oman, D., Thoresen, C. E., & McMahon, K. (1999). Volunteerism and mortality among the community-dwelling elderly. *Journal of Health Psychology, 4,* 301-316.

Pargament, K. I. (1997). *The psychology of religion and coping: Theory, research, practice.* New York: The Guilford Press.

Pargament, K. I., Ensing, D. S., Falgout, K., Olsen, H., Reilly, B., Van Haitsma, K., & Warren, R. (1990). God help me (I): Religious coping efforts as predictors of the outcomes to significant negative life events. *American Journal of Community Psychology, 18,* 793-824.

Pargament, K. I., Koenig, H. G., & Perez, L. M. (2000). The many methods of religious coping: Development and initial validation of the RCOPE. *Journal of Clinical Psychology, 56,* 519-543.

Pargament, K. I., Olsen, H., Reilly, B., Falgout, K., Ensing, D. S., & Van Haitsma, K. (1992). God help me (II): The relationship of religious orientations to religious coping with negative life events. *Journal for the Scientific Study of Religion, 31* 504-513.

Pargament, K. I., Smith, B. W., Koenig, H. G., & Perez, L. (1998). Patterns of positive and negative religious coping with major life stressors. *Journal for the Scientific Study of Religion, 37,* 710-724.

Park, C. L., & Cohen, L. H. (1993). Religious and nonreligious coping with the death of a friend. *Cognitive Therapy and Research, 17,* 561-577.

Park, C. L., Cohen, L. H., & Murch, R. L. (1996). Assessment and prediction of stress-related growth. *Journal of Personality, 64,* 71-105.

Prigerson, H. G., Bierhals, A. J., Kasl, S. V., Reynolds, C. F., Shear, M. K., Newsom, J. T. & Jacobs, S. (1996). Complicated grief as a disorder distinct from bereavement-related depression and anxiety: A replication study. *American Journal of Psychiatry, 153,* 1484-1486.

Prigerson, H. G., Frank, E., Kasl, S. V., Reynolds, C. F., Anderson, B., Zubenko, G. S., Houck, P. R., George, C. J., & Kupfer, D. J. (1995). Complicated grief and bereavement-related depression as distinct disorders: Preliminary empirical validation in elderly bereaved spouses. *American Journal of Psychiatry, 152,* 22-30.

Princeton Religious Research Center (1994). Importance of religion. *PRRC emerging trends, 16,* 4.

Richards, A., & Folkman, S. (1997). Spiritual aspects of bereavement among partners of men who died of AIDS. *Death Studies, 21,* 527-552.

Sanders, C. M. (1981). Comparison of younger and older spouses in bereavement outcome. *Omega, 11,* 217-232.

Sanders, C. M. (1993). Risk factors in bereavement outcome. In M. S. Stroebe, W. Stroebe, & R. O. Hansson (Eds.), *Handbook of bereavement research: Theory, research, and intervention* (pp. 256-267). Cambridge: Cambridge University Press.

Schaefer, C., Quesenberry, C. P., Jr., & Wi, S. (1995). Mortality following conjugal bereavement and the effects of a shared environment. *American Journal of Epidemiology, 141*, 1142-1152.

Scheier, M. F., Weintraub, J. K., & Carver, C. S. (1986). Coping with stress: Divergent strategies of optimists and pessimists. *Journal of Personality and Social Psychology, 51*, 1257-1264.

Schultz, R., Beach, S. R., Lind, B., Martire, L. M., Zdaniuk, B., Hirsch, C., Jackson, S., & Burton, L. (2001). Involvement in caregiving and adjustment to death of a spouse: Findings from the caregiver health effects study. *Journal of the American Medical Association, 285*, 3123-3129.

Seltzer, M. (1976). Suggestions for the examination of time-disordered relationships. In J. F. Gubrium (Ed.), *Time, roles, and self in old age* (pp. 111-125). New York: Human Sciences Press.

Sonnenblick, M., Friedlander, Y., & Steinberg, A. (1993). Dissociation between the wishes of terminally ill parents and decisions by their offspring. *Journal of the American Geriatrics Society, 41*, 599-604.

Stein, N., Folkman, S., Trabasso, T., & Richards, T. A. (1997). Appraisal and goal processes as predictors of psychological wellbeing in bereaved caregivers. *Journal of Personality and Social Psychology, 72*, 872-884.

Stroebe, M. (1992). Coping with bereavement: A review of the grief work hypothesis. *Omega, 26*, 19-42.

Stroebe, M., Gergen, M. M., Gergen, K. J., & Stroebe, W. (1992). Broken hearts or broken bonds: Love and death in historical perspective. *American Psychologist, 47*, 1205-1212.

Stroebe, W., & Schut, H. (2001). Risk factors in bereavement outcome: A methodological and empirical review. In M. S. Stroebe, R. O. Hansson, W. Stroebe, & H. Schut (Eds.), *Handbook of bereavement research: Consequences, coping, and care* (pp. 349-371). Washington, DC: American Psychological Association.

Stroebe, W., & Stroebe, M. S. (1987). *Bereavement and health.* New York: Cambridge University Press.

Stroebe, M. S., & Stroebe, W. (1993). *Handbook of bereavement; Theory, research and intervention.* Cambridge: Cambridge University Press.

Tait, R., & Silver, R. C. (1989). Coming to terms with major negative life events. In J. S. Uleman & J. A. Bargh (Eds.), *Unintended thought* (pp. 351- 382). New York: Guilford.

Tedeschi, R., & Calhoun, L. (1996). The Post-Traumatic Growth Inventory: Measuring the positive legacy of trauma. *Journal of Traumatic Stress, 9*, 455-471.

Thompson, L. W., Gallagher-Thompson, D., Futterman, A., Gilewki, M. J., & Peterson, J. (1991). The effects of late-life spousal bereavement over a 30-month interval. *Psychology and Aging, 6*, 434-441.

Troll, L. E. (1986). *Family issues in current gerontology.* New York: Springer.

US Bureau of the Census (2000). Marital Status and living arrangements: March 2000. *Current Population Reports*. Washington, DC: US Government Printing Office.

Wheaton, B. (1990). Life transitions, role histories, and mental health. *American Sociological Review, 55*, 209-223.

Worden, J. W. (1991). *Grief counseling and grief therapy: A handbook for the mental health practitioner*. New York: Springer.

Wyatt, G. K., Friedman, L., Given, C. W., & Given, B. A. (1999). A profile of bereaved caregivers following provision of terminal care. *Journal of Palliative Care, 15*, 13-25.

Zisook, S., & Shuchter, S. R. (1993). Major depression associated with widowhood. *The American Journal of Geriatric Psychiatry, 1*, 316-326.

Not on Their Own Again: Psychological, Social, and Health Characteristics of Custodial African American Grandmothers

Dorothy S. Ruiz, PhD
Carolyn W. Zhu, PhD
Martha R. Crowther, PhD, MPH

SUMMARY. The article presents social and health indicators of depression among custodial African American grandmothers. Using a cross-sectional design, a sample of 99 custodial African American grandmothers caring for one or more grandchildren was included in the analysis. The results indicated that approximately 20% of custodial African American grandmothers were depressed. Depressed grandmothers were more likely to report having all ten chronic physical health conditions listed in the

---

Address correspondence to: Dorothy S. Ruiz, PhD, Department of African American and African Studies, 9201 University City Boulevard, University of North Carolina at Charlotte, Charlotte, NC 28223 (E-mail: dsruiz@email.uncc.edu).

This manuscript was supported by the Duke University Center for the Study of Aging and Human Development, The National Institutes of Health, National Institute on Aging, Physiology in Aging Account No. 2T32AG00029 and The National Institute on Aging Account No. R01 AG 15062-03S1.

[Haworth co-indexing entry note]: "*Not* on Their Own Again: Psychological, Social, and Health Characteristics of Custodial African American Grandmothers." Ruiz, Dorothy S., Carolyn W. Zhu, and Martha R. Crowther. Co-published simultaneously in *Journal of Women & Aging* (The Haworth Press, Inc.) Vol. 15, No. 2/3, 2003, pp. 167-184; and: *Widows and Divorcees in Later Life: On Their Own Again* (ed: Carol L. Jenkins) The Haworth Press, Inc., 2003, pp. 167-184. Single or multiple copies of this article are available for a fee from The Haworth Document Delivery Service [1-800-HAWORTH, 9:00 a.m. - 5:00 p.m. (EST). E-mail address: docdelivery@haworthpress.com].

10.1300/J074v15n02_10

study. One additional chronic condition increased the probability of depression by 68%. Old age, more social support, and caring for older children were associated with low levels of depression. The proliferation of grandchildren being raised by African American grandmothers suggests the need for more research, policy, and programmatic interventions.

[Article copies available for a fee from The Haworth Document Delivery Service: 1-800-HAWORTH. E-mail address: <docdelivery@haworthpress.com> Website: <http://www.HaworthPress.com> © 2003 by The Haworth Press, Inc. All rights reserved.]

KEYWORDS. Grandparents, caregivers, grandchildren, kinship care, surrogate parents

There has been increased attention on the number of grandchildren living in homes headed by grandparents in the past two decades. This trend began as early as the 1970s. According to the Census Bureau (1992), the number of children under 18 living in grandparent-maintained households increased from 2.2 million in 1970, to 2.3 million in 1980, to 3.3 million in 1992. In 1970, slightly more than 3 percent of all children under 18 were living in a home headed by a grandparent. This number had increased to almost 5 percent by 1992. Recent research and census data show that this trend continued through the 1990s. In 1997, for example, 3.9 million children lived in a home maintained by a grandparent, consisting of 5.5 percent of all children under 18 years old (Bryson and Casper, 1999). Significant increases have occurred in the number of children living with grandparents where only one or no biological parent is present (Bryson and Casper, 1999). Between 1970 and 1992, the greatest increase was among grandchildren living with grandparents with only one parent present. However, between 1992 and 1997, the greatest increase has occurred among grandchildren living with grandparents with no biological parent present (Bryson and Casper, 1999).

The majority of grandparents who live with grandchildren are grandmothers. In 1997, among the 4.7 million grandparents who were living with grandchildren, 2.9 million (62%) were grandmothers (Bryson and Casper, 1999). Grandmothers often provide care for their grandchildren as a result of family crises involving the parents of the grandchildren, such as drug use, unemployment, teenage pregnancy, divorce, abuse and neglect, abandonment, and death. More recent societal problems, such as acquired immunodeficiency syndrome (AIDS) (Lesar, Gerber, and Simmel, 1995; Le Blanc, London, and Aneshensel, 1997) and incarcerations of the parents (Barnhill, 1996; Dressel and Barnhill, 1994; Gaudin, 1984) are additional reasons for grandmothers to care for their grandchildren. The striking increase in children being raised by grandparents because of their parents' substance abuse, incarcerations, and AIDS has led to unanticipated long-term care responsibility. These and other contemporary social problems have prompted researchers to investigate the relationship between custodial grandparenting and psychological distress (Bowers and Myers, 1999; Burnette, 1999; Burton, 1992; Emick and Hayslip, 1996; Kelley, 1993; Kelley et al., 2000; Minkler and Roe, 1993; Minkler, Roe, and Price, 1992; Minkler et al., 1997; Roe, Minkler, and Barnwell, 1994; Sands and Goldberg-Glen, 1996; Shore and Hayslip, 1994; Strawbridge et al., 1997; Szinovacz, DeViney, and Atkinson, 1999). In spite of the increased interest in the topic over the last two decades, there is a scarcity of information on the impact of caregiving on the psychological well-being of custodial African American grandmothers. This article will examine the relationships between social factors, health status, and depression among custodial African American grandmothers.

BACKGROUND

Existing literature has identified some factors that affect depression among grandparents. In their analysis of the second wave of the National Survey of Families and Households, Minkler, Fuller-Thomson, Miller, and Driver (1997), found that depressive symptoms were associated with caring for a grandchild. Other factors found to be associated with low levels of depression included older age, higher family income, greater number and better quality of social networks, being married, and being in excellent health. Although Minkler and associates (1997) found an inverse relationship between age and depression, suggesting that grandmothers over 65 seem to be more comfortable with the grandparenting role than younger grandmothers, results from other studies found the relationship between age and depression is not clear (Blazer, Burchett, Service, and George, 1991; Raymond and Michaels, 1980).

Among African American grandmothers, age may have different effects on depression. In African American communities, older women caring for grandchildren and other relatives is not uncommon (Billingsley,

1992). Many have taken care of young relatives for all of their adult life. However, younger grandmothers may not be comfortable with the grandmother roles because of competing factors, including employment, competing family demands, active social life, or the need to be involved with their own minor children. There has been little research that examines the associations between custodial caregiving and the onset of depression among African American grandmothers.

Studies have shown that the demands of custodial caregiving among grandparents may affect physical health as well (Burnette, 1999; Minkler and Roe, 1993; Minkler, Roe, and Price, 1992; Minkler and Fuller-Thomson, 1999; Musil, 1998). In their exploratory study of physical and emotional health of 71 African American grandmothers raising their grandchildren because of crack-cocaine use of the parents, Minkler, Roe, and Price (1992) found that 44% of the respondents were in pain; 49% had back pain; and 25% had heart trouble. Slightly over one-third of the grandmothers reported that their health worsened after assuming care of their grandchildren. Musil (1998), on the other hand, in a small study of 90 grandmothers, including both Whites and Blacks, found no differences in physical and emotional health between grandmothers who were primary caregivers and those who were not. To date, results on the relationship between custodial grandparenting and grandmothers' physical health are inconclusive. Even less is known about this relationship among African American grandmothers.

The relationship between social support and depression in later life is well established in the literature (Aneshensel, Frerichs, and Huba, 1984; George, 1992; Szinovacz, DeViney, and Atkinson, 1999). However, the relationship between social support and depression among caregiving grandmothers is less clear. Only a few studies have addressed how the quality and number of supports for grandparent caregivers affect their psychological health (Burnette, 1999; Minkler and Roe, 1993; Poe, 1992; Musil, 1998); most of these are the results of qualitative approaches. The general consensus is that support for grandparents is limited (Burnette, 1999; Minkler and Roe, 1993; Musil, 1998). Musil (1998) found that custodial grandmothers reported receiving less instrumental and subjective support than non-custodial grandmothers did. Research on the importance of social support on the current generation of African American grandmothers is sketchy at best.

This paper will provide insight into relationships between selected social and health variables, and depression among custodial African American grandmothers. The following questions will be addressed: What are the social, demographic, and physical health characteristics of custodial grandmothers? Is depression associated with age of grand-mother, age of grandchildren, physical health, and social support?

METHODS

Sample

A cross-sectional research design was used to examine demographic characteristics, physical health, and psychological well-being among African American grandmothers who were primary caregivers for at least one grandchild. The study population consisted of 99 custodial African American grandmothers who resided in the Triangle and Piedmont areas of North Carolina. Grandmothers who were eligible for the study must have met the following criteria: (1) was the primary caregiver for one or more grandchildren or great-grandchildren under age 18; (2) was non-institutionalized; (3) resided in the Triangle or Piedmont areas of North Carolina; and (4) viewed herself as being in a permanent grand-parenting relationship with the grandchild.

Data Collection

Five North Carolina counties were involved in the study. These included Durham, Guilford, Mecklenburg, Orange, and Wake counties. A number of organizations and persons provided assistance in identifying grandmothers who met the study criteria: North Carolina Division on Aging, Durham County Social Services, Durham County Housing Authority, Orange County Housing Authority, senior centers support groups, community nurses, mental health centers, family social workers in public schools, and juvenile detention facilities were among the agencies involved. Representatives from the above agencies were asked to help identify grandmothers within their agencies who were custodial caregivers for at least one grandchild in the defined geographical areas. The study also used word of mouth recruitment through local African American churches, cultural community organizations, and grandparent participants. After a list of grandmothers had been identified, those who expressed an interest in the study were pre-screened to determine their eligibility for inclusion. Once the inclusion criteria were satisfied, an appointment was made by the principal investigator to meet with the grandparent at a location convenient to the subject. Most of the interviews took place in the subjects' homes, with the exception of a few who were interviewed at support group meetings.

The data collection instrument was pre-tested using a focus group of 10 grandmother caregivers to eliminate any difficult questions and to make the protocol more understandable and relevant to this sample. All interviews were conducted by the principal investigator (first author) between June 1999 and October 2000. Most interviews took from 2 to 3 hours each to complete. However, occasionally, an interview might take as long as 4 or 5 hours depending on the openness and personality of the grandmother. This was the only opportunity for some grandmothers to discuss their experiences and vent their differences and frustrations. In a few cases, where the interview was interrupted or became too extensive, a follow-up interview was scheduled or completed over the telephone. These were instances where the grandchild may have returned from school and needed the attention of the grandmother. Or, the grandchild's parent may have entered the interview setting and the grandmother did not wish to discuss her childcare burden in their presence. The demanding work schedules of some grandmothers made telephone interviews necessary.

Measures

The instrument consisted of approximately 350 questions seeking primarily quantitative information, and approximately 30 questions seeking qualitative information. All survey instruments were approved by the Institutional Review Board of Duke University Medical Center. The major issues in the questionnaire included the following 12 components: demographic characteristics, household composition, economic resources, family competing demands, reasons for providing care, church and social support, value orientation and family relationships, religiosity, physical health and chronic conditions, life satisfaction, depression, and stress symptoms. In this paper, we focus on the effects of demographic and social characteristics and physical health on depression.

Demographic and social characteristics. Demographic characteristics included age, education, marital status, employment status, family income, sources of income, wealth, religion, social support, and household composition. Household composition was measured by the number and age of grandchildren the grandmother cared for, years of care provision, and whether an adult lived in the grandmother's household.

Physical health. This measure consisted of a list of physical health conditions that might affect the grandmother (Brown and Monye,

1995). The chronic conditions included arthritis, cancer, stroke, diabetes, problems breathing, high blood pressure, circulation problems, heart problems, glaucoma, and kidney disease.

Depression. Depressive symptomatology was measured by a modified version of the Center for Epidemiological Studies Depression Scale (CES-D) (Radloff, 1977). There were no changes in the content of the questions. All questions from the CES-D were included in their original version. However, instead of the original scale that measured each question in a 0-3 scale, the modified response categories were combined into a yes/no format for reporting the presence or absence of a symptom during the week preceding the interview. The revised instrument has been tested extensively by Duke University investigators (Blazer, Burchett, Service, and George, 1991) to determine its comparability to the original CES-D Scale. Their results indicate that the modified instrument was virtually identical to the original instrument.

Previous studies have shown that a score of 16 or higher on the original scale represents clinically significant depressive symptoms (Radloff, 1977). Blazer et al. (1991) showed that a score of 9 or greater on the revised scale was equivalent to the score of greater than or equal to 16 on the original scale. Accordingly, we constructed a dichotomous variable that equals to 1 to indicate depression if the total CES-D score equaled to 9 or greater and 0 if the score was less than 9 to indicate the absence of depressive symptoms.

Social support. The measure of social support used in this study was the number of people grandmothers could rely on for help. This consisted of four different categories of social and emotional support. Subjects were asked to list all individuals they could depend on in each category, and indicate their level of satisfaction.

Analysis

We examined sociodemographic and physical health characteristics of grandmothers who had depressive symptomatology (reported total CES-D score greater than or equal to 9) and grandmothers who were not depressed (reported total CES-D score less than 9) separately. Student t-tests were used to test for differences in means in the continuous variables and chi-squared tests were used for discrete variables. A logistic regression was performed to examine the effects of sociodemographic and physical health characteristics on depressive symptomatology of the grandmothers. STATA program was used for computations (STATA, 1994).

RESULTS

Table 1 shows social and demographic characteristics of the 99 grand-mothers included in this study, by grandparents' depressive symptom-atology. The grandmothers ranged in age from 38 to 88, with an average age of 58. Eight percent of the sample were younger than 45; 66% were 45-74 years old; 20% were between 65-74; and 6% were 75 and older. The average grandmother in the sample had finished 11.5 years of schooling. Thirty-six percent were high school graduates and 38% did not finish high school. Almost three-quarters of the grandmothers (74%) were not married and were heads of household. The other 26% lived with their spouses. Although only a quarter of the grandmothers in this sample were 65 and older, more than half (51%) were retired. Twenty-nine percent of the sample were employed full-time and 9% were employed part-time. The remaining 9% who reported that they were neither employed nor retired were grandmothers who had never been in the paid workforce.

The average family income of this sample of African American grand-mothers was $21,100, with a median income at $17,500. Eleven percent of the grandmothers in the sample had household incomes below $5,000; 22% had incomes between $5,001-10,000; 24% between $10,001-20,000; 15% between $20,001-30,000; 11% between $30,001-40,000; and 16% greater than $40,000. The higher incomes were associated with married grandmothers, or grandmother-maintained households consisting of employed adult children. Many grandmothers received their incomes from multiple sources. Fifty-four percent of the grandmothers received their incomes from wages and salaries, 43% from social security, 15% from disability payments, 23% from retirement pensions, 13% from Supplemental Security Income (SSI), and 38% from Welfare pay-ments/Work First. Six percent of their incomes came from relatives or other sources. Close to 57% owned their own homes, and 16% reported owning other real estate property. Most of the homeowners lived in mo-bile homes in rural North Carolina. We did not ask the grandmothers to enumerate their wealth holdings.

Religion is very important to older African American women. In the African American community, elderly women are considered the back-bone of the church as well as the family. More than 50% of the sample were Baptist (56%), 11% were Methodist, 25% reported to be affiliated with other religions, including Catholic, Lutheran, Muslim, Pentecos-tal, Presbyterian, and Holiness. Only a small number of grandmothers in the sample were not church members (8%). However, regardless of

Table 1. Sociodemographic Characteristics of African-American Caregiving Grandmothers (n = 99)

Variable	All sample	Depression Status	
		Not depressed	Depressed
	Mean (s.d.)	Mean (s.d.)	Mean (s.d.)
N	99	80	19
Mean CES-D score	4.5 (5.0)	2.4 (2.4)	13.3 (2.9)
Age (mean years)*	57.6 (10.1)	58.6 (10.3)	53.3 (7.5)
Younger than 45 (%)	8.1	7.5	10.5
45-54 (%)	35.4	32.5	47.4
55-64 (%)	30.3	28.8	36.8
65-74 (%)	20.2	23.8	5.3
75 or older (%)	6.1	7.5	0.0
Years of schooling completed	11.5 (2.6)	11.6 (2.2)	11.2 (3.8)
Less than high school (%)	38.4	37.5	42.1
High school graduate (%)	36.4	37.5	31.6
Some college (%)	21.2	21.3	21.1
College graduate (%)	4.0	3.8	5.3
Marital status (%)			
Married	26.3	28.8	15.8
Divorced/separated	40.4	36.3	57.9
Widowed	22.2	25.0	10.5
Never married	11.1	10.0	15.8
Employment status (%)			
Retired	51.5	50.0	57.9
Full time	29.3	30.0	26.3
Part time	9.1	7.5	15.8
Not employed	9.1	11.3	0
Other	3.0	2.5	5.3
Family income in 1998 ('000 $)	21.1 (16.0)	21.6 (1.7)	19.1 (4.2)
Median ('000 $)	17.5	17.5	12.5
Less than $5,000	11.1	8.8	21.1
$5,001-$10,000	22.2	21.3	26.3
$10,001-$15,000	15.2	16.3	10.5
$15,001-$20,000	9.1	10.0	5.3
$20,001-$30,000	15.2	15.0	15.8
$30,001-$40,000	11.1	13.8	0.0
Greater than $40,000	16.2	15.0	21.1

TABLE 1 (continued)

| | | Depression Status | |
Variable	All sample	Not depressed	Depressed
N	Mean (s.d.)	Mean (s.d.)	Mean (s.d.)
Sources of Income (%)	99	80	19
Wages and salaried	53.5	55.0	47.4
Social security (Excluding SSI) *	43.4	50.0	15.8
Disability payments*	15.2	11.3	31.6
Retirement pension	23.2	23.8	21.1
Supplemental Security Income	13.1	15.0	5.3
Welfare payments/Work first	38.4	35.0	52.6
Wealth (%)			
Own home	56.6	60.0	42.1
Own any other real estate	16.2	17.5	10.5
Religion (%)			
Baptist	55.6	57.5	47.4
Methodist	11.1	12.5	5.3
No religion	8.1	7.5	10.5
Other religion	25.3	22.5	36.8
Number of people can rely on	1.8 (1.3)	1.9 (1.3)	1.1 (0.9)
Number of grandchildren*	2.0 (1.4)	1.8 (1.3)	2.5 (1.7)
One (%)	47.5	50.0	63.2
Two or more (%)	52.5	50.0	36.8
Age of grandchild*	7.9 (5.2)	8.5 (5.2)	5.4 (4.5)
5 or younger	17.2	15.0	26.3
6-11	45.5	43.8	52.6
12-17	29.3	31.3	21.1
18 or older	8.1	10.0	0
Years of caring for grandchild	7.3 (4.8)	7.7 (4.8)	5.7 (4.7)
Two or fewer	24.2	21.3	36.8
3-9	42.4	42.5	42.1
10 or more	33.3	36.3	21.1
Has coresident adult child (%)	33.3	36.3	21.1
Age of coresident adult child	32.2 (7.8)	31.9 (9.1)	33.2 (7.2)

Notes:
Standard deviations are shown in parentheses.
Child refers to the grandmothers' adult child.
* Difference between depressed and non-depressed grandmothers statistically significant at
0.05 level.

church membership, all grandmothers said that their spiritual beliefs were very important in providing care for their grandchildren.

On average, the grandmothers in this sample cared for 2 grandchildren for about 7 years. The average age of the custodial children was 8 (range 6 months to 25 years old); almost half (46%) were between age 6 and 11. Only a third of the grandmothers reported having a co-resident adult child. The average age of coresident adult children was 32 years.

Table 1 also shows social and demographic characteristics for grandmothers who had depressive symptoms (CES-D score greater than or equal to 9) and compared them with those who did not (CES-D score less than 9). The majority of the custodial grandmothers in this sample (80%) were not depressed, with an average CES-D score of 2.4). Those who were depressed reported an average CES-D score of 13.3 (s.d. = 2.9). Lower CES-D scores were significantly associated with older ages (p = .03), not receiving social security benefits (p = .007), receiving disability payments (p = .03), having a greater number of social supports (p = .01), having more custodial grandchildren (p = .02), and caring for older grandchildren (p = .02). There is a trend toward significance between depression and being divorced or separated (p = .08), high income (p = .09), and fewer years of custodial care provision (p = .09). No associations were found in the bivariate analysis for high school completion, employment status, home ownership, religious participation, years of caregiving, and having at least one coresident adult child.

Table 2 presents bivariate results of physical health status of the custodial grandmother by their depressive symptomatology. Grandmothers who were depressed (having CES-D score 9 or greater) on average had three chronic conditions, one more than grandmothers who were not depressed (p = .03). Two-thirds of all grandmothers had high blood pressure and about half had arthritis. Grandmothers who were depressed were more likely to report having all ten conditions inquired about in the survey. The differences in the probability of reporting each of the following diseases was tremendous: Grandmothers who were depressed were more than twice as likely to report problems with breathing (47% vs. 20%, p = .01), almost three times as likely to report glaucoma (37% vs. 13%, p = .01), more than twice as likely to report heart problems (32% vs. 14%, p = .07), more than four times as likely to report cancer (21% vs. 5%, p = .02), and more than five times as likely to report kidney disease (21% vs. 4%, p = .008). Possibly because of the small sample, rates of high blood pressure, arthritis, circulation problems, diabetes, and stroke were not significantly different between these two groups.

TABLE 2. Physical Health Status of African-American Caregiving Grandmothers (n = 99)

Variable	All sample	Depression Status	
		Not depressed	Depressed
	Mean (s.d.)	Mean (s.d.)	Mean (s.d.)
N	99	80	19
Number of chronic conditions*	2.2 (1.6)	2.1 (1.5)	3.0 (1.8)
High blood pressure	61.6	61.3	63.2
Arthritis	44.4	42.5	52.6
Problem with breathing*	25.3	20.0	47.4
Diabetes	25.3	23.8	31.6
Circulation problems	22.2	20.0	31.6
Heart problems	17.2	13.8	31.6
Glaucoma*	17.2	12.5	36.8
Cancer*	8.1	5.0	21.1
Stroke	8.1	6.3	15.8
Kidney disease*	7.1	3.8	21.1

Notes:
Standard deviations are shown in parentheses.
* Difference between depressed and non-depressed grandmothers statistically significant at 0.05 level.

A logistic regression was performed to determine the relationship between grandparent caregiving and depression, controlling for sociodemographic factors that have been found to be associated with depressive symptoms (Table 3). The outcome variable is 1 if the grandmother was depressed (CES-D score greater or equal to 9), and 0 if not depressed (CES-D score less than 9). The model is highly significant (p < .001). Consistent with results from the bivariate analyses, older age (p < .05), more social support (p < .05), and caring for older children (p < .05) are all associated with low levels of depression. Indeed, having one more person the grandmother can rely on for help decreased the probability of her being depressed by 41%. Not surprisingly, depression was associated with an increased number of chronic conditions (p < .0001): Having one more chronic condition increased the probability of being depressed by 68%. Unfortunately, the size of the sample precluded an analysis of the effects of individual conditions separately. Neither high

TABLE 3. Predictors of Depression (CES-D Score Greater Than or Equal to 9) Among African-American Caregiving Grandmothers (n = 99)

Variables	Coefficient	Standard error	Odds ratio
Age 65 or older = 1	−2.028**	1.177	0.13
Less than high school education = 1	−0.388	0.683	0.68
Married or widowed = 1	−0.666	0.657	0.51
Number of chronic conditions	0.521***	0.193	1.68
Number of people can rely on	−0.527**	0.279	0.59
Age of youngest grandchild	−0.138**	0.071	0.87
Constant	−0.128	0.905	
Prob > χ^2	0.0004		

Note: * significant at 10% level; ** significant at 5% level, *** significant at 1% level.

school completion nor marital status was associated with depression in the logistic regression analysis.

FUTURE DIRECTIONS

The purpose of this study is to make a contribution to the existing research on the impact of social and health factors on custodial African American grandmothers. In spite of the nonrandom, self-selected sample, we believe the results contribute to a better understanding of the experiences of African American grandmothers who are primary caregivers.

A bivariate analysis comparing depression scores for selected demographic variables showed low depression scores among grandmothers who were older, married, and had high incomes. Low depression scores were also associated with grandmothers who received social security benefits, had more social support and who cared for older children. In a logistic regression, age, social support, and caring for older children continued to be associated with low levels of depression. High depression scores were associated with increased numbers of chronic health conditions.

Differences in depressive symptomatology by grandmothers' marital status is of note. The majority of the grandmothers in this sample were widowed, or divorced/separated. In our bivariate analysis, a larger proportion of widows were depressed but a smaller proportion of divorced/separated grandmothers were. While data revealed a trend toward significance between depression and being divorced/separated, the difference was no longer significant after controlling for other factors. It appears that in this group of custodial grandmothers, not being married does not have any ill effects in terms of grandmothers' psychological well-being.

The findings from this study are consistent with previous studies showing high rates of depression among women (George, 1995; Beckman, 1995; Minkler, Fuller-Thomson, Miller, and Driver, 1997). The lower depression scores among older grandmothers is consistent with findings from Minkler et al. (1997). Conflicting role responsibilities are often associated with young grandmothers who may be employed or have minor children of their own.

All but a few grandmothers in the sample stated that they felt overwhelmed by responsibility. Burton (1992) found that grandparents frequently requested respite care from parenting. However, out of guilt that they might have failed as parents and out of fear that child protective services might remove the children from their care, African American grandmothers are often reluctant to seek opportunities for a break. In comparison to younger grandmothers, older African American grandmothers report feeling less overwhelmed by responsibility, and their attitudes about caregiving are generally more approving. Older grandmothers place caregiving of any kind at the forefront of their existence. The sacrifices they make for their children and grandchildren are central to their belief system concerning their roles as women and their devotion to children.

The lack of informal support was common among these grandmothers. Although some studies have suggested that the traditional extended family network in African American communities is an important source of social support (Billingsley, 1992; Hill, 1997; Martin and Martin, 1985), grandmother caregivers in this study received little support from family and friends. Grandmothers relied heavily on their faith, and often cited God as their only source of support. Only 2 of the 99 grandmothers in the sample reported receiving help in some form from the African American church. George et al. (1989) found that high levels of social support are associated with decreased levels of psychiatric morbidity, particularly depression.

This study has identified several areas for future research. The circumstances under which grandmothers assume care of their grandchildren have not been researched well. We believe that research on this issue would broaden our understanding of the transition from parental care to grandparent care. More information is needed concerning the level of knowledge grandparents have with respect to providing care at different stages of the grandchild's social and emotional development. Although many similarities exist among African American and White custodial grandmother caregivers, many differences are found (Fuller-Thomson, Minkler, and Driver, 1997; Szinovacz, 1998). The meaning of caregiving across racial and ethnic groups suggests different needs for research and program development. Research on the impact of social support on African American grandmothers is sketchy.

This study is particularly meaningful in that African American grandmothers are as diverse in their socioeconomic characteristics as they are in attitudes about caregiving and their styles of delivering care. While some enjoy the challenge, many feel trapped and obligated, others clearly resent the role. More research and programs need to address the resentment that African American grandmothers feel as a result of being primary caregivers. The traditional meaning of the social support network has clearly broken down in African American communities. The high volume of support that Black families once received is no longer available to grandmothers.

Several limitations must be considered concerning this sample of grandmother caregivers. Although it is a small, purposive, self-selected, nonrandom sample, we believe that it is a fairly good representation of custodial grandmothers in African American communities. Given the cross-sectional nature of the data, causal attributions are not possible. Longitudinal studies are needed to determine the prevalence of depression, and its impact on caregiving as well as the caregiver. This sample included only grandmothers who were mobile, with few debilitating problems. We do not know what differences there might be among caregivers who are less mobile, and with more severe health conditions. The sample does not represent a broad range of education and occupational differences. However, in spite of the limitations, there are specific characteristics in this sample which have similarities to national data (Bryson and Casper, 1999; Fuller-Thomson, Minkler, and Driver, 1997; Szinovacz, 1998).

This paper has provided a clearer picture of the social, psychological, and physical characteristics of African American grandmothers who are custodial caregivers. Program and policy agenda must address the need to support families headed by single African American grandmothers who have special problems and unusual circumstances. They are at a time in life when they might have expected to be "on their own again," without the child-rearing responsibilities associated with earlier life stages. Grandmothers who do not have a spouse due to death, divorce, or separation would especially expect to be relatively free from family responsibilities. In spite of these expectations, we see that many African American grandmothers take on the demands of caring for young children, often in the face of ill health and reduced social support.

There is a need for support services for grandmothers, particularly respite care. A relatively new program seeks to address some of this need: Under the Older American's Act, states can use National Family Caregiver Support Program (NFCSP) funds to provide services such as respite care for grandmother caregivers (65 and older) of children under 18 years of age. In addition, perhaps policymakers should consider extending NFCSP eligibility to younger grandmothers, or providing funds for a similar program for younger grandmothers. Younger grandmothers are experiencing more depression which is likely due to multiple demands on their time since many are still working. Respite care, a primary service offered through NFCSP, may be more important to their well-being than to older grandmothers. Policy makers and practitioners must develop policies and programs that assist grandparent caregivers to continue providing for their grandchildren by building strong family units and to cope with the demands of caregiving that can adversely affect their physical and psychological well-being.

REFERENCES

Aneshensel, C., Frerichs, R., & Huba, G. (1984). Depression and physical illness: A multiwave, nonrecursive model. *Journal of Health and Social Behavior, 25,* 350-371.

Barnhill, S. (1996). Three generations at risk: The imprisoned women, their children, and the grandmother caregiver. *Generations, 20*(1), 39(2).

Beckman, E., & Leber, W. (1995). *Handbook of depression* (2nd. ed.). New York: NY Press.

Billingsley, A. (1992). *Climbing Jacobs Ladder: The enduring legacy of African American families.* New York: Simon and Schuster.

Blazer, D., Burchett, B., Service, C., & George, L. (1991). The association of age and depression among the elderly. An epidemiologic exploration. *Journal of Gerontology, 46*(6), M210- 215.

Bowers, B., & Myers, B. (2000). Grandmothers providing care for grandchildren: Consequences of various levels of caregiving. *Family Relations, 48*(3), 303-311.

Brown, D. R., & Monye, D. B. (1995). *Midlife and older African Americans as intergenerational caregivers of school-aged children.* AARP Andrus Foundation

Final Report. Research Information Center, 601 E. Street NW, Room B3-1, Washington, DC 20049.

Bryson, K., & Casper, L. (1999). *Co-resident grandparents and grandchildren.* U. S. Census Bureau, Current Population Reports, Special Studies, pp. 23-198, Washington, DC.

Burnette, D. (1999). Physical and emotional well-being of custodial grandparents in Latino families. *American Journal of Orthopsychiatry, 69*(3), 305-318.

Burton, L. M. (1992). Black grandparents rearing children of drug-addicted parents: Stressors, outcomes and social service needs. *The Gerontologist, 32*(6), 744-751.

Dressel, P., & Barnhill, S. (1994). Reframing gerontological thought and practice: The case of grandmothers with daughters in prison. *The Gerontologist, 34,* 685-690.

Emick, M., & Hayslip, B. (1996). Custodial grandparenting: New roles for middle aged and older adults. *International Journal of Aging and Human Development, 43*(2), 135-154.

Fuller-Thomson, E., Minkler, M., & Driver, D. (1997). A profile of grandparents raising grandchildren in the United States. *The Gerontologist, 37*(3), 406-411.

George, L. K., Blazer, D. G., & Hughes, D. C. et al. (1989). Social support and the outcome of major depression. *British Journal of Psychiatry, 154,* 478-485.

George, L. K. (1992). Social factors and the onset and outcome of depression. In K.W. Schaie, J. S. House, & D. G. Blazer (Eds.), *Aging, health behaviors and health outcomes* (pp. 137-159). Hillsdale, NJ: Lawrence Erlbaun Associates.

George, L. (1995). Social factors and illness. In Binstock R. H., Gerorge, L. K. (Eds.), *Handbook of aging and the social sciences* (4th ed.). New York, NY: Academic Press Inc.; 229-252.

Gaudin, T. M. (1984). Social work roles and tasks of incarcerated mothers. *Social Casework, 65*(5), 279-286.

Hill, R. (1997). *The strengths of African American families: Twenty-five years later.* Washington, DC: R & C Publishing.

Kelley, S., Whitley, D., Sipe, T., & Yorker, B. (2000). Physical distress in grandmother kinship care providers: The role of resources, social support, and physical health. *Child Abuse and Neglect, 24*(3), 311-321.

Kelley, S. J. (1993). Caregiver stress in grandparents raising grandchildren. *Journal of Nursing Scholarship, 25*(4), 331-337.

LeBlanc, A., London, A., & Aneshensel, C. (1997). The physical costs of AIDS caregiving. *Social Science and Medicine, 45*(6), 915-923.

Lesar, S., Gerber, M., & Simmel, M. (1995/96). HIV infection in children: Family stress, social support and adaptation. *Exceptional Children, 62*(3), 4-236.

Martin, E. P., & Martin, J. M. (1985). *The helping tradition in the Black family and the community.* Silver Spring, MD: NASW.

Minkler, M., & Fuller-Thomson, E., Miller, D., & Driver, D. (1997). Depression in grandparents raising grandchildren. *Archives of Family Medicine, 6,* September, 445-452.

Minkler, M., Fuller-Thomson, E. (1999). The health of grandparents raising grandchildren. Results of a national study. *American Journal of Public Health, 89,* 1384-1389.

Minkler, M., Roe, K., & Price, M. (1992). The physical and emotional health of grandmothers raising grandchildren in the crack-cocaine epidemic. *The Gerontologist, 32,* 752-760.

Minkler, M., & Roe, K. (1993). *Grandmothers as caregivers. Raising children of the crack-cocaine epidemic.* Newbury Park, CA: Sage.

Musil, C. (1998). Health, stress, coping, and social support in grandmother caregivers. *Health Care for Women International, 19,* 441-455.

Poe, L. (1992). Black grandparents as parents. Library of Congress: 516-580.

Raymond, E., & Michaels, T. (1980). Prevalence of correlates of depression in elderly persons. *Psychological Reports, 47,* 1055-1061.

Radloff, L. S. (1977). CES-D Scale: A Self-Report Depression Scale for research in a general population. *Applied Psychological Measurement, 3,* 385-401.

Roe, K., Minkler, M., & Barnwell, R. (1994). The assumption of caregiving: Grandmothers raising the children of the crack-cocaine epidemic. *Qualitative Health Research, 4*(3), 281-303.

Sands, R. G., & Goldberg-Glen, R. S. (1996). *The impact of surrogate parenting on grandparents: Stress, well-being, and life satisfaction.* AARP Andrus Foundation Final Report. Research Information Center, 601- E. Street NW, Room B3-1, Washington, DC 20049.

Shore, R. J., & Hayslip, J. B. (1994). Predictors of well-being in custodial and non-custodial grandparents. Boston: Paper presented at American Psychological Association.

Strawbridge, W. J., Wallhagen, M. I., Shema, S. J., & Kaplan, G. A. (1997). New burdens or more of the same? Comparing grandparent, spouse, and adult child caregivers. *Gerontologist, 37*(4), 505-510.

STATA StataCorp. (1994). Stata Statistical Software: Release 6.0. College Station, TX, Stata Corporation.

Szinovacz, E. S., DeViney, S., & Atkinson, M. P. (1999). The effects of surrogate parenting on grandparents' well-being. *Journal of Gerontology, 54B*(6), S376-388.

Szinovacz, M. E. (1998). Grandparents today: A demographic profile. *The Gerontologist, 38*(1), 37-52.

U.S. Bureau of the Census. (1992). Census of the Population. *Marital Status and Living Arrangements.* Current Population Reports, Population Characteristics, Series P-20, No. 468, Washington, DC: U.S. Government Printing Office, March 1992.

Conclusions

Carol L. Jenkins, MPA, PhD

This volume presents new perspectives on the lives of older widows and divorcees, and on some of the problems they face in adjusting to and living life without a spouse. The theme of women on their own again was chosen to address the perception that older widows and divorcees are on their own again because they have lost a spouse. As the authors of various articles have made clear, in reality most older widows and divorcees are not on their own again, but live within specific social and cultural networks from which they receive a great deal of support.

Perhaps one of the most important issues facing older widows and divorcees is coping with loss. While all have lost a spouse, they are often dealing with other losses as well: independence, financial security, and social and instrumental support, to name a few. Michael, Crowther, Schmid, and Allen stress the importance of religion and spirituality when used as coping methods for dealing with loss. Religion is an important means of coping with other life problems as well, as shown by Ruiz, Zhu, and Crowther. They identify the significance of religious faith to custodial African American grandmothers, some of whom state that it is their only means of support.

Social support is one of the more important forms of support for older widows and divorcees, and several authors have addressed this. Laditka and Laditka show that maintaining social connections with family members, friends, and neighbors helps to overcome the adverse health

[Haworth co-indexing entry note]: "Conclusions." Jenkins, Carol L. Co-published simultaneously in *Journal of Women & Aging* (The Haworth Press, Inc.) Vol. 15, No. 2/3, 2003, pp. 185-187; and: *Widows and Divorcees in Later Life: On Their Own Again* (ed: Carol L. Jenkins) The Haworth Press, Inc., 2003, pp. 185-187. Single or multiple copies of this article are available for a fee from The Haworth Document Delivery Service [1-800-HAWORTH, 9:00 a.m. - 5:00 p.m. (EST). E-mail address: docdelivery@haworthpress.com].

10.1300/J074v15n02_11

effects related to the death of a spouse. Social support is associated with lower levels of depression for custodial African American grandmothers as shown by Ruiz, Zhu, and Crowther. Reduced levels of depression, in turn, are associated with better health; thus, social support has positive effects on both psychological and physical well-being.

Children play a major role in providing both social and instrumental support to mothers, helping to alleviate the ill effects of widowhood and divorce. Jenkins shows that children's willingness and ability to provide informal assistance can prevent their widowed mother's admission to institutionalized care and help them remain in their own homes in the face of a great deal of physical disability. Both McNally and Cattell emphasize the importance of family, and particularly adult child, support for older widowed mothers in non-Western countries. Lacking such support, many widows would find themselves in dire circumstances. Family support appears to have greater importance in developing nations because of lower public support in the form of social welfare policies.

While we have seen that many older widows and divorcees are doing relatively well, not all are. Some lack social and instrumental support and are essentially on their own again. Lacking family support, they often find themselves alone in the community, struggling to maintain their physical and economic viability. Or, they are compelled to seek publicly funded community services or institutionalized care. Glaser, Grundy, and Lynch identify the recent trend of older widows and divorcees in Great Britain to move to institutionalized care rather than moving into coresidence with family or other supportive adults. Angel, Douglas, and Angel show that widows are more likely to use community-based services, while widowers tend to enter nursing homes when their health has deteriorated. At the same time, widows face greater financial strains and are more dependent on public programs such as Supplemental Security Income and Medicaid.

Economic security is of great importance to older women. Adequate income can fill in the gaps to some extent when social support is lacking. Butrica and Iams look at a future cohort of older divorcees who might be expected to be better off than the current cohort, at least in terms of economic well-being. They predict, not surprisingly, that women in the baby boom cohort who are better educated, own a home, and have pension and asset income will be better off financially. These characteristics are more likely to be found in baby boom women due to the increased opportunities they faced in their lifetimes for education and labor market participation. At the same time, not all women have had equal opportunities for education and good jobs. Black and Hispanic women are less likely to have a college education, own a home, or have pension and asset income. Thus, older Black and Hispanic divorcees are likely to have lower retirement incomes and to face economic insecurity.

We need to remember those older widows and divorcees who are lacking family and social networks; they tend to be the oldest, poorest, and most disabled, and are dependent to a great extent on the community's good will. It is these women who most need assistance from the public policy and private charitable sectors. At the same time, it is clear that the perception that older widows and divorcees are on their own again is not accurate for many women. While they have lost a spouse, they have a wide range of supports, including social contacts with and instrumental help from family and friends, strong religious beliefs, and social policies intended to enhance their physical, psychological, and economic well-being. They truly are not "on their own again."

About the Contributors

Rebecca S. Allen, PhD, is Assistant Professor, Department of Psychology, and Associate Director, Applied Gerontology Program, University of Alabama. Her research program concerns interventions to improve quality of life and the process of health care decision making for older adults and their families. Specific research interests include interventions to improve communicative interactions regarding advance care planning between health care professionals, older adults, and personal caregivers in palliative and long-term care settings; improving access to palliative care and hospice for ethnically diverse patient/caregiver dyads and for those with end-stage neurodegenerative disorders; and the factors underlying the relation between personal and proxy health care decisions, including cultural perceptions of quality of life.

Jacqueline L. Angel, PhD, is Associate Professor at the LBJ School of Public Affairs and Faculty Research Affiliate of the Center for Health and Social Policy, The University of Texas at Austin. In 1990-92, she was NIA Postdoctoral Fellow in the Demography of Aging Training Program at Pennsylvania State University. Angel has written on a number of social policy issues related to health and minority aging with a special emphasis on Hispanic populations. She is particularly interested in how cultural heterogeneity among the elderly affects the design of programs for the cost-effective delivery of acute and long-term care. Her participation in the H-EPESE project has involved a study of the impact of nativity and migration processes on health outcomes, and their implications for care and living arrangements.

Ronald J. Angel, PhD, received his degree from the University of Wisconsin-Madison, and has been a member of the faculty of the University of Texas at Austin since 1991. His research interests encompass the areas of medical sociology, social welfare, poverty and minorities, demography and epidemiology, research methods, and statistics. Recent books, with Jacqueline L. Angel, are *Who Will Care for Us? Aging and Long-Term*

http://www.haworthpress.com/store/product.asp?sku=J074
© 2003 by The Haworth Press, Inc. All rights reserved.
10.1300/J074v15n02_12

Care in Multicultural America, New York: New York University Press (1997) and *Painful Inheritance: Health and the New Generation of Fatherless Families*, Madison, WI: University of Wisconsin Press (1993).

Barbara A. Butrica, PhD, is a Research Associate in the Urban Institute's Income and Benefits Policy Center. Her research interests are in the fields of labor economics, public finance, poverty, and demography. Of particular interest are issues related to the study of aging and income dynamics. She is currently involved in a number of projects that assess the impact of Social Security retirement and survivors, programs on the economic security of the aged.

Maria G. Cattell, PhD, anthropologist and Research Associate at The Field Museum of Natural History, has taught at Franklin and Marshall College, Lebanon Valley College, and Millersville University. Her research focuses on older people and social change, families, intergenerational relationships, gender and power. She has been doing long-term research among Abaluyia in Kenya since 1982 and has also carried out research among Zulus in South Africa and with older white ethnics in Philadelphia. She is co-author with Steven Albert of *Old Age in Global Perspective: Cross-Cultural and Cross-National Views* (G.K. Hall, 1994) and co-editor with Jacob Climo of *Social Memory and History: Anthropological Perspectives* (AltaMira, 2002). Currently she is co-editing a volume of the personal and professional narratives of women who received their PhDs in anthropology from the age of 45 up.

Martha R. Crowther, PhD, is Assistant Professor, Department of Psychology and Faculty Scholar, Center for Mental Health and Aging, University of Alabama. Her research interests are focused on clinical geropsychology, with a primary interest in the nature, impact and consequences of custodial grandparenting as well as designing effective interventions to reduce stress in this population. Additionally, she has explored the relation between spirituality and mental health across the life span and cultural diversity in research and clinical training.

Nora Douglas is a master's candidate in the Department of Sociology at the University of Texas at Austin. Her research interests include aging, long-term care, and evaluation research. Her master's thesis investigates the high turnover rates among the paraprofessional workforce and possible effects of stress and coping on job satisfaction.

Karen Glaser, BA, MA, MSc, PhD, a demographer, is Lecturer in Gerontology and Programme Organiser for the MSc in Gerontology at the Age Concern Institute of Gerontology (ACIOG), King's College, London. Her main research interests are in comparisons of co-residence, kin availability, proximity, and the provision of care between older people in Britain and Southern Europe; the living arrangements of older people in Britain and changes in residence patterns over time; the complex inter-relationships between the multiple roles of mid-life individuals in Britain, focusing on work and family commitments, and how they may affect quality of life in old age; and social class differences in the provision of care among those in mid-life in Britain.

Emily Grundy, BA, MSc, PhD, a demographer, is Reader in Social Gerontology and Head of the Centre for Population Studies, London School of Hygiene and Tropical Medicine, where she leads the annual short course on *Ageing, Health and Well-Being in Older Populations.* Her main research interests are in health, disability and mortality, particularly at older ages, and in families, households and kin and social networks, especially in relationship to health. Much of her research has used data from the Office for National Statistics Longitudinal Study and she is leader of the Centre for Longitudinal Study Information and User Support programme.

Howard M. Iams, PhD, received his degree in sociology from the University of Michigan. He is a Social Science Research Analyst in the Office of Research, Evaluation, and Statistics, Social Security Administration, Washington, DC. For the past twenty years, he has been working with surveys matched to Social Security Administration records. He has worked on the development of the MINT data system with SIPP matched to Social Security Administration records for the past six years.

James N. Laditka, DA, PhD, is Research Assistant Professor, Department of Epidemiology and Biostatistics, Arnold School of Public Health, University of South Carolina. His research focuses on health care use and health disparities associated with race and ethnicity, income, and insurance status. His research has been published in numerous journals.

Sarah B. Laditka, PhD, is Associate Professor, Department of Health Administration, Arnold School of Public Health, University of South Carolina. Her research focuses on utilization, access, and quality of health services for vulnerable populations, use of formal and informal long-term care services, and the quality of older life and active life expectancy for older populations. Dr. Laditka's research has been published in numerous journals. She is the editor of *Health Expectations of Older Women: International Perspectives.*

Kevin Lynch, BSc, holds a degree in computer science from Trinity College in Dublin. He is Senior LS Support Officer with the Longitudinal Study Development Unit at the Office for National Statistics. He previously worked with the LS Support Programme at the Centre for Longitudinal Studies, Institute of Education. Currently he is working on developing the ONS Longitudinal Study databases and preparing for the linkage of data from the 2001 Census.

James W. McNally, PhD, is Director of the National Archive of Computerized Data on Aging (NACDA) at the Institute for Social Research at the University of Michigan. He has worked on aging research in both the United States and internationally in the Pacific and Asia and has an ongoing interest in issues related to family care of elders. The paper presented in this volume is an outgrowth of work initiated in the Philippines as part of a larger project funded by the MacArthur Foundation and was supported by funding from the National Institute on Aging (P30AG004590).

Scott T. Michael, PhD, is Postdoctoral Fellow at the VA Medical Center, Seattle, Washington. He received his degree in clinical psychology from the University of Kansas where he studied the role that hope plays in facilitating adaptive coping to stressful and traumatic life events such as bereavement. His fellowship research is focused on PTSD in the veteran population at the VA Puget Sound Health Care System.

Dorothy S. Ruiz, PhD, is Associate Professor, Department of African American and African Studies, University of North Carolina at Charlotte. Her research interests are role-stress relationships among grandmother caregivers in intergenerational families, African American family history, and the social psychology of health and aging. The focus of her current research is the "health and social indicators of stress among African American grandmothers who are primary caregivers in intergenerational families." Her research has appeared in numerous journals; a major contribution is *The Handbook of Mental Health and Mental Disorder Among Black Americans.*

Bettina Schmid, MA, is a graduate student in the clinical psychology program at the University of Alabama. Her research interests are in the area of health psychology. Currently she is working on dissertation research, studying end-of-life medical decision making among older adults. She is a licensed professional counselor with over ten years of clinical experience and has served as the executive director of a community-based organization serving people affected by HIV/AIDS.

Carolyn W. Zhu, PhD, is a Senior Research Associate at the Robert J. Milano Graduate School of Management and Urban Policy, New School University. She received a PhD in economics from Duke University and was an NIH Fellow at the Center for the Study of Aging and Human Development at Duke University. Her fields of study include applied econometrics and health economics, with a focus on older people.

Index

ACIOG. *See* Age Concern Institute of
    Gerontology (ACIOG)
Activities of daily living (ADLs), 9,
    128
ADLs. *See* Activities of daily living
    (ADLs)
Affleck, G., 154-155
African widows, 49-67
    problems and concerns of, 57-61
    sociodemographic overview of,
        50-51
    socioeconomic and cultural
        contexts of widowhood
        among, 54-57
    transformations among, colonial
        and postcolonial, 52-54
    true story of, 50
Age, as factor in widowhood, 146-148
Age Concern Institute of Gerontology
        (ACIOG), King's College,
        London, 190-191
AIMEs. *See* Average indexed monthly
        earnings (AIMEs)
Albert, S., 190
Allen, R.S., 5,145,159,185,189
Andersen, R.M., 11
Angel, J.L., 5,89,186,189
Angel, R.J., 5,89,189-190
Aranda, M.P., 103
Auxiliary beneficiary, defined, 74-75
Average indexed monthly earnings
        (AIMEs), 74
Aykan, H., 11

Baby boomers, divorced female,
        67-88. *See also* Divorcee(s),
        older; Divorcee(s), retired;
        Retiree(s), divorced

projected retirement income of,
        minority group status effects
        on, 67-88
    introduction to, 68-70
    at retirement, 71,71t
Beneficiary
    auxiliary, defined, 74-75
    dually entitled, 75
    retired-worker, 75-76
Bereavement
    conjugal, 146
    coping responses to, 145-165
        future directions in, 158-160
    definitions related to, 146, 150-151
    described, 146
    physical health and, 149
    psychological well-being in,
        148-149
    religion and, 150-151
    religious coping and, 150-151,
        153-158
    social support in, 149
    spirituality and, 150-151
    terminal care services use and,
        149-150
Blazer, D., 173
BMI. *See* Body mass index (BMI)
Body mass index (BMI), 15
Bourgeois, M., 159
Bowen, E.S., 32
Bower, J.E., 154
Bulman, J., 152
Burgio, L.D., 159
Burica, B.A., 67
Burton, L.M., 180
Butrica, B.A., 186,190
Byles, J., 9,10

193

Cain, M., 31
Caregiving, as factor in widowhood, 148
Carnelley, K.B., 148
Carr, D., 24
Cattell, M.G., 4,49,186,190
Census Bureau, 168
Center for Epidemiological Studies Depression Scale (CES-D), 95,173
Center for Health and Social Policy, University of Texas–Austin, 189
Centre for Population Studies, London School of Hygiene and Tropical Medicine, 191
CES-D. *See* Center for Epidemiological Studies Depression Scale (CES-D)
Chaplin, W.F., 159
Chyba, M.M., 11
Climo, J., 190
Cochran-Mantel-Haenszel test, 21
Coffey, R.M., 15
Community Care Act, 124
Community-based services, 95
Conceptual model of hospitalization, for recently widowed older women, 11-14
    enabling factors for, 12-13
    need factors for, 13-14
    predisposing factors for, 12
    social contacts and, 14
Conjugal bereavement, 146
Coping, religious
    in bereavement adjustment, 150-151,152-158
    defined, 150-151
    life stressors and, 152-158
Cowgill, D.O., 31
Crowther, M.R., 5,145,167,185,186, 190
Custodial African American grandmothers
    prevalence of, 168

psychological, social, and health characteristics of, 167-184
    historical background of, 169-171
    study of
        analysis of, 173-174
        data collection in, 171-172
        future directions in, 179-182
        measures in, 172-173
        methods in, 171-173
        results of, 174-179,175t-176t, 178t,179t
        sample in, 171

Davis, C.G., 155
Days Since Last Discharge, 24
DeLaine, S., 159
Demography of Aging Training Program, at Pennsylvania State University, 189
Dijkstra, K., 159
Divorcee(s)
    baby-boomer, projected retirement income of, minority group status effects on, 67-88
    baby-boomer, projected retirement income of, minority group status effects on. *See also* Baby boomers, divorced female, projected retirement income of, minority group status effects on
    in later life, 4-5
        introduction to, 1-7
    older
        economic well-being of, 2
        in England and Wales, transitions to supported environments in, 107-126
            analysis plan, 114-115
            introduction to, 108-110
            multivariate analysis of, 119-122,120t,122t
            study data, 110-115

study discussion, 122-124
study methods, 110-115
study results, 115-116, 15t
terminology related to,
          111-112
transitions to supported
          private households
          and institutions in,
          117-119,118t
type of independent/
          supported private
          household at end of
          interval in, 116-117,
          116t
focus on, 2-4
living arrangements of, 3
physical health of, 3
psychological well-being of, 3
social support of, 3-4
retired
     beneficiary status of, 74-77,75t,
          76t,78f,79f
     demographic characteristics of,
          71t,72-74,72t
     income of, 78-79,80f,81t
     demographic and socioeconomic
          effects on, 79-83, 82t
     minority gap in, accounting for,
          83-84,83t
Douglas, N., 5,89,186,190
Driver, D., 169
Dually entitled beneficiary, 75
Duke University, 173,192
Duke University Medical Center,
          Institutional Review Board
          of, 172
Durham County Housing Authority,
          171
Durham County Social Services, 171

Economic well-being, of older widows
          and divorcees, 2
Elderly

divorced, in England and Wales,
          transitions to supported
          environments in, 107-126.
          See also Divorcee(s), older,
          in England and Wales,
          transitions to supported
          environments in
Mexican-American, gender,
          widowhood, and long-term
          care in, 89-105. *See also*
          Mexican American
          population, older, gender,
          widowhood, and long-term
          care in
widowed
     care arrangement choices for,
          127-143. *See also* Widow(s),
          older, care arrangement
          choices for
     in England and Wales,
          transitions to supported
          environments in, 107-126.
          See also Widow(s), older, in
          England and Wales,
          transitions to supported
          environments in
Elixhauser, A., 15
England, transitions to supported
          environments among elderly
          widowed and divorced
          women, 107-126. *See also*
          Divorcee(s), older;
          Widow(s), older

Family(ies), defined, 111
Family households, defined, 111
Feldman, S., 9, 10
Fiji, health, widowhood, and family
          support in, study of, 29-47
     background of, 31-32
     data from, 33-36,34t
     discussion of, 43,45-46
     introduction to, 30
     methodology in, 32-36,34t

multivariate analysis model in, 36
research sites in, 32-34
results of, 37-43,38t,39t,41f,42f,44f
Fitti, J.E., 11
Franklin and Marshall College, 190
Frantz, C.M., 155
Freeman, V.A., 11
Freud, S., 158
Friedlander, Y., 159
Friedman, L., 148
Fuller-Thomson, E., 169

George, L.K., 152,180
Gergen, K.J., 158
Gergen, M.M., 158
Gilbar, O., 152
Given, B.A., 148
Given, C.W., 148
Glaser, K., 5, 107,186,190-191
Goldman, N., 9,10,24
Grandmother(s), custodial African
American. *See* Custodial
African American
grandmothers
Grundy, E., 5,107,186,191

Hansson, R.O., 147
Harris, R., 15
Health care, home, defined, 95
Health characteristics, of custodial
African American
grandmothers, 167-184. *See
also* Custodial African
American grandmothers,
psychological, social, and
health characteristics of
*Health Expectations of Older Women:
International Perspectives,*
191
Health maintenance organizations
(HMOs), 11
H-EPESE. *See* Hispanic Established
Populations for

Epidemiological Studies of
the Elderly (H-EPESE);
Longitudinal Study of elderly
Mexican American Health
Hispanic Established Populations for
Epidemiological Studies of
the Elderly (H-EPESE), 94
Hispanics. *See* Mexican American
population
HMOs. *See* Health maintenance
organizations (HMOs)
Home health care, defined, 95
Hospitalization, for recently widowed
older women, 7-28. *See also*
Widow(s), in later life,
increased hospitalization risk
for
Household(s)
family, defined, 111
independent, defined, 113
private
defined, 111
supported, defined, 113
Howard, A., 32

IADLs. *See* Instrumental activities of
daily living (IADLs)
Iams, H.M., 67,186,191
Income, of divorced retirees, 78-79,
80f, 81t
Independence, maintaining of, family's
importance in, 137-138
Independent households, defined, 113
Institute for Social Research,
University of Michigan,
National Archive of
Computerized Data on Aging
at, 192
Institution(s), defined, 112-113
Institutional Review Board of Duke
University Medical Center,
172
Instrumental activities of daily living
(IADLs), 128

Jacobs, S., 147, 148
Janoff-Bulman, R., 155
Jenkins, C.L., 1, 127, 185
Johnson, R.J., 11-12

Kasl, S.V., 147
Kelly, B., 149
King's College, London, Age Concern
    Institute of Gerontology at,
    190-191
Koenig, H.G., 150,152,155
Koreman, S., 9
Kovar, M.G., 11

Laditka, J.N., 4,7,185,191
Laditka, S.B., 4,7,185,191
Larson, D.B., 150
Larson, J., 149, 156
Lebanon Valley College, 190
Life stressors, religious coping and,
    152-158
Lillard, L.A., 10
Living arrangements, of older widows
    and divorcees, 3
London School of Hygiene and
    Tropical Medicine, Centre for
    Population Studies at, 191
Longitudinal Study of Aging (LSOA),
    8,9,11,14,15,24
Longitudinal Study of Elderly Mexican
    American Health
    (H-EPESE), 89, 94
LSOA. *See* Longitudinal Study of
    Aging (LSOA)
Lynch, K., 5,107,186,191-192

MacArthur Foundation, 192
Major Diagnostic Categories (MDCs),
    21,22t
Marital status, of retirees, 71,71t
Marson, D.L., 159
Martin, L.G., 11,31
Marwit, S.J., 146

Matthews, S.H., 138
McCorkle, R., 149-150
McCullough, M., 150
McIntosh, D.N., 154
McMahon, K., 157
McNally, J.W., 4,29,186,192
MDCs. *See* Major Diagnostic
    Categories (MDCs)
Medicaid, 89,186
Medicare, 11,19
Mendes de Leon, C.F., 147
Mexican American population, older,
    gender, widowhood, and
    long-term care in, 89-105
    historical background of, 92-94
    introduction to, 90-91
    study of
        data from, 94-96
        discussion of, 101-103
        measures in, 94-96
        methods in, 94-96
        results of, 96-101,96t,98t-101t
Michael, S.T., 5,145,185,192
Miller, D., 169
Millersville University, 190
Mini Mental Status Exam (MMSE), 95
Minkler, M., 169,170,180
MINT. *See* Modeling Income in the
    Near Term (MINT)
MINT data system, 70
Mishra, G., 9
MMSE. *See* Mini Mental Status Exam
    (MMSE)
Modeling Income in the Near Term
    (MINT)
    described, 70-71
    SSA's, 67,70
Moskowitz, J.T., 154
Moss, M.S., 147
Moss, S.Z., 147
Musil, C., 170

NACDA. *See* National Archive of
    Computerized Data on Aging
    (NACDA)

National Archive of Computerized
Data on Aging (NACDA), at
Institute for Social Research,
University of Michigan, 192
National Family Caregiver Support
Program (NFCSP), 182
National Health Service (NHS), 124
National Institute on Aging, 192
National Long Term Care Survey, 102
National Survey of Families and
Households, 169
Nesse, R., 24
New School University, Robert J.
Milano Graduate School of
Management and Urban
Policy of, 192
NFCSP. *See* National Family
Caregiver Support Program
(NFCSP)
NHS. *See* National Health Service
(NHS)
1988 National Survey of Hispanic
Elderly People, 93
Nolen-Hoeksema, S., 149,156
Nonbeneficiary, 76
defined, 74
North Carolina Division on Aging, 171
Nursing facility use, defined, 96

Office for National Statistics (ONS)
Longitudinal Study (LS),
108,110-111
*Old Age in Global Perspective:
Cross-Cultural and
Cross-National Views,* 190
Older Americans Act, 25
Oman, D., 157
ONS Longitudinal Study. *See* Office
for National Statistics (ONS)
Longitudinal Study (LS)
Orange County Housing Authority,
171

Painful Inheritance, 190
Palawan, in Phillipines, health,
widowhood, and family
support in, study of, 29-47.
See also Phillipines, health,
widowhood, and family
support in, study of
Panapasa, S., 32
Panel Study of Income Dynamics
(PSID), 70
Pargament, K.I., 150,151,156-157
Pennsylvania State University,
Demography of Aging
Training Program at, 189
Perez, L.M., 152
Phillipines, health, widowhood, and
family support in, study of,
29-47
background of, 31-32
data from, 33-36,34t
discussion of, 43,45-46
introduction to, 30
methodology in, 32-36,34t
multivariate analysis model in, 36
research sites in, 32-34
results of, 37-43,38t,39t,41f,42f 44f
Physical health
as factor in widowhood, 149
of older widows and divorcees, 3
PIA. *See* Primary insurance amount
(PIA)
Potash, B., 55,56,59
Price, M., 170
Primary insurance amount (PIA), 74,
75-76,77
Private households
defined, 111
supported, defined, 113
PSID. *See* Panel Study of Income
Dynamics (PSID)
Psychological characteristics, of
custodial African American
grandmothers, 167-184. *See
also* Custodial African
American grandmothers,

psychological, social, and
health characteristics of
Psychological well-being
as factor in widowhood, 148-149
of older widows and divorcees, 3

RCOPE, 152,153
Reciprocity, in care arrangement
choices for older widows,
138-139
Religion, bereavement and, 150-151
Religious coping
as acquisition of social support,
156-157
in bereavement adjustment,
150-151,152-158
defined, 150-151
life stressors and, 152-158
as maintaining bond to deceased,
157-158
Religious coping scale (RCOPE), 152,
153
Rensal, J., 32
Responsibility, in care arrangement
choices for older widows,
138-139
Retired-worker beneficiary, 75-76
Retiree(s)
divorced
beneficiary status of, 74-77,75t,
76t,78f,79f
demographic characteristics of,
71t,72-74,72t
income of, 78-79,80f,81t
demographic and
socioeconomic
effects on, 79-83,
82t
minority gap in, accounting
for, 83-84,83t
marital status of, 71,71t
Retirement income, projected, of
divorced female baby
boomers, minority group
status effects on, 67-88

Robert J. Milano Graduate School of
Management and Urban
Policy, New School
University, 192
Roe, K., 170
Rosner, T.T., 138
Ruiz, D.S., 5,167,185,192

Safety issues, care arrangement
choices for older widows,
137
SAS GENMOD procedure, 18
Schaefer, C., 149
Schmid, B., 5,145,185,192
Schuchter, S.R., 148
Schultz, R., 148
Schut, H., 149
Senior service, defined, 95-96
Siegler, I.C., 152
Silver, R.C., 154
SIPP. *See* Survey of Income and
Program Participation (SIPP)
SMSAs. *See* Standard Metropolitan
Statistical Areas (SMSAs)
Social characteristics, of custodial
African American
grandmothers, 167-184. *See
also* Custodial African
American grandmothers,
psychological, social, and
health characteristics of
*Social Memory and History:
Anthropological
Perspectives,* 190
Social Security Administration (SSA),
MINT of, 67, 70
Social Security benefits, 1,2,68,78,80f
Social Security disability insurance
(DI), 70
Social support
as factor in widowhood, 149
of older widows and divorcees, 3-4
religious coping as acquisition of,
156-157

Socioeconomic factors, effects on
     income of divorced retirees,
     79-83,82t
Sonnenblick, M., 159
Spirituality
     bereavement and, 150-151
     widowhood and, 145-165. *See also*
          Widowhood, spirituality and
SSA. *See* Social Security
          Administration (SSA)
SSI. *See* Supplemental Security
          Income (SSI)
SSI program. *See* Supplemental
          Security Income (SSI)
          program
Standard Metropolitan Statistical
          Areas (SMSAs), 13, 14
STATA program, 173
Steinberg, A., 159
Steiner, C., 15
Stressor(s), life, religious coping and,
          152-158
Stroebe, M., 149
Stroebe, W., 158
Supplemental Security Income (SSI),
          186
Supplemental Security Income (SSI)
          program, 85
Survey of Income and Program
          Participation (SIPP), 70

Tait, R., 154
Tennen, H., 154-155
Terminal care services, as factor in
          widowhood, 149-150
The Handbook of Mental Health and
          Mental Disorder Among
          Black Americans, 192
Thoresen, C.E., 157
Torres, M.S., 103
Trinity College, Dublin, 191-192

Umberson, D., 10

University of Alabama, 189,190,192
University of Michigan, 191
     National Archive of Computerized
          Data on Aging at Institute for
          Social Research at, 192
University of North
          Carolina–Charlotte, 192
University of South Carolina, 191
University of Texas–Austin, 189,190
     Center for Health and Social Policy
          at, 189
University of Wisconsin–Madison, 189
Urban Institute's Income and Benefits
          Policy Center, 190
U.S. Physician Payment Review
          Commission, 13
Utz, R.L., 24

VA Medical Center, Seattle,
          Washington, 192
VA Puget Sound Health Care System,
          192
Vanua Levu, in Fiji, health,
          widowhood, and family
          support in, study of, 29-47.
          See also Fiji, health,
          widowhood, and family
          support in, study of
Vlassoff, C., 31

Waite, L.J., 10
Wales, transitions to supported
          environments among elderly
          widowed and divorced
          women, 107-126. *See also*
          Divorcee(s), older;
          Widow(s), older
Weinstein, R., 9
Well-being
     economic, of older widows and
          divorcees, 2
     psychological
          as factor in widowhood, 148-149

of older widows and divorcees,
3
WHA. *See* Women's Health Australia
(WHA)
Wheaton, B., 148
*Who Will Care for Us? Aging and
Long-Term Care in
Multicultural America,*
189-190
Widow(s)
African, 49-67. *See also* African
widows
increased hospitalization risk for,
introduction to, 8-9
older, 4-5
care arrangement choices for,
127-143
discussion of, 139-142
family's importance in
maintaining
independence in,
137-138
historical background of,
128-130
maintaining woman's
independence in,
133-136
reciprocity in, 138-139
responsibility in, 138-139
safety concerns in, 137
study of
data analysis in, 133
data collection in, 131
methods in, 130-133,132t
results of, 133-139
sample in, 131-133,132t
sample selection in,
130-131
economic well-being of, 2
in England and Wales,
transitions to supported
environments in, 107-126
analysis plan, 114-115
introduction to, 108-110

multivariate analysis of,
119-122,120t, 122t
study data, 110-115
study discussion, 122-124
study methods, 110-115
study results, 115-116,115t
terminology related to,
111-112
transitions to supported
private households
and institutions in,
117-119,118t
type of independent/
supported private
household at end of
interval in,
116-117,116t
focus on, 2-4
increased hospitalization risk
for, 7-28
study of
conceptual model
development in,
11-14
data from, 11
discussion of, 23-26
hazard models in, 16-18
methods in, 11-18
policy implications of,
23-26
results of,
18-23,18t,20t,22t
variable coding in, 14-16
introduction to, 1-7
living arrangements of, 3
physical health of, 3
psychological well-being of, 3
social contacts of, protective
effects of, 7-28
introduction to, 8-9
social support of, 3-4
risk of being, 8
Widowhood
age as factor in, 146-148
caregiving in, 148

in Fiji, study of, 29-47. *See also*
    Fiji, health, widowhood, and
    family support in, study of
issues impacting experience of,
    146-150
in Phillipines, study of, 29-47. *See
    also* Phillipines, health,
    widowhood, and family
    support in, study of
physical health in, 149
psychological well-being in,
    148-149
social support in, 149
spirituality and, 145-165

future directions in, 158-160
terminal care services use and,
    149-150
transition to, 9-11
Within Two-Year Bereavement Period,
    19-20
Wolinsky, F.D., 11
Women's Health Australia (WHA), 9
Worden, J.W., 157
Wortman, C.B., 24,152
Wyatt, G.K., 148

Zhu, C.W., 5,167,185,186,192
Zisook, S., 148